Optimal Nutrition for Cancer Patients

A Comprehensive Dietary Plans for Enhancing Your Body's Natural Power to Healing while Working with Your Doctor for Maximum Recovery

Johanne M. Martinez

Disclaimer

The author and publisher disclaim any liability or responsibility to any person or entity for any loss or damage caused, or alleged to be caused, directly or indirectly, by the information contained in this book.

Dedication

To the brave souls navigating the stormy seas of cancer treatment, may this book serve as a lighthouse, guiding you to the safe harbor of health and well-being.

Remember, like broccoli, you are both tough and beneficial. May your spirits stay as unshakable as a well-rooted carrot, and your laughter as infectious as a contagious calorie.

This book is dedicated to every patient, caregiver, and healthcare warrior. May you find strength in these pages and humor in the face of adversity.

If kale had muscles, it'd be flexing for you right now!

TABLE OF CONTENTS

Introduction

Life Story: You can beat cancer again

I always thought life was simple: finish your homework, play your favorite sport, go to bed, repeat. Easy peasy. I was living in an illusion, blissfully unaware of the miracles and tragedies life can throw at you in the blink of an eye. One day, I got a harsh reality check.

I believed I was living my finest life. I woke up, got ready, and headed to school, but something felt off. Maybe it was the cafeteria food catching up with me, or perhaps my body was plotting against me. Nonetheless, I attended every lecture and had a pretty decent day. I didn't mention anything to my family and acted like my usual, healthy self.

A week went by, and I finally decided to spill the beans to my mom. I told her I was feeling weird, like my body had a mind of its own. She shared this with my dad, who's a doctor. He handed me some tablets and sent me to bed.

The next morning, I was still in dreamland when I felt my mom's hand on my stomach, probably checking if I was turning into a superhero overnight. Instead, she felt something strange.

My stomach felt like it was auditioning for a role in a rock band. She freaked out and called my dad, who decided we needed a hospital visit.

Two hours of poking and prodding later, the doctor suggested we head to another city for better treatment. My parents, voices trembling, asked, "Another city? Why? What's going on, Doctor?"

The doctor dropped the bombshell: "Your daughter shows symptoms of a serious disease. I suspect its cancer." The ground slipped from under their feet. Tears flowed, questions flew, and the doctor, clearly in a hurry, excused himself, leaving us in a sea of confusion and fear.

That was our first serious family crisis. Everyone was speechless, and I began to struggle with even the simplest tasks. Moving, walking, and climbing into bed became Herculean efforts. Finally, we got an answer: ***Tata Memorial Hospital in Mumbai***. We had to leave within two days. It was the second stage of ovarian cancer, and tension hung heavy in the air.

That night, I saw my father crying like never before. I wanted to comfort him, but I was too weak. Seeing him weep broke my heart, and I couldn't hold back my own tears.

It was our worst day ever. I didn't know much about cancer, only that it was a one way ticket to somewhere scary.

"Cancer? How long do I have?" I asked, feeling as if I were in a horrible movie. The doctor explained it was the end of the second stage, and it had spread. I barely understood, but my dad's face said it all. Papers were signed, and soon I was in the operating theater. Miraculously, the surgery was successful.

You can't imagine that phase. I'll tell you more about it another time. Just when I thought it couldn't get worse, I had exams coming up. The doctor said I couldn't leave the hospital, but I insisted. I had to take my board exams. He refused initially, but after a lot of pleading, he allowed me to go home for the exams.

I aced them, scoring a respectable first division. My dad, expecting 95+, wasn't thrilled, but given the circumstances, I think I did pretty well. I became a source of inspiration for my schoolmates, proving that even in the face of cancer, I could still achieve my goals.

Cancer taught me many lessons. It took away one of my ovaries but gave me a new perspective on life. I realized that cancer could touch my body but never my mind, heart, or soul. Life is about accepting challenges and proving yourself. It's simple, really – don't make it complicated.

I've faced many hard times and have many more years to live, but I'm grateful for the experience. It helped me unleash my hidden potential. Life is about exploring and learning. If you're not growing, you're missing out. You may blend in or stand out; the option is yours.

I love traveling and meeting new people and documenting my journey into writing. Every month, I explore new places and cultures. Cancer showed me the true colors of people, even those closest to me. Life is a rollercoaster with ups and downs, and I'm facing every phase with grace. Despite being a cancer patient, I dream big and give my all to every moment.

Life is about living in the now and chasing dreams.

Difficulties are just opportunities to uncover your hidden strength. If I can survive cancer and achieve my dreams, so can you. Believe in yourself, and you will overcome any challenge.

Part 1:
Understanding the Foundation

Chapter 1: The Biology of Cancer: An Overview

Imagine your body as a meticulously conducted orchestra. Each cell, a skilled musician, plays its part in harmony, following a precise score – the genetic instructions encoded in our DNA. This intricate performance sustains life, growth, and repair. But what happens when a rogue conductor disrupts the harmony, rewriting the score and leading the orchestra into a cacophony of uncontrolled growth? This, in essence, is the essence of cancer.

Cancer is not a single disease, but rather a constellation of over 200 distinct conditions, each arising from a complex interplay of genetic mutations and environmental factors. At the core of this transformation lies a breakdown in the finely tuned communication system that governs cellular behavior. Normally, our cells meticulously follow a preprogrammed script: grow, divide, and die in a controlled manner. This ensures the orderly renewal of tissues and organs while maintaining a healthy balance.

However, cancer cells become akin to rebellious musicians, ignoring the conductor's cues and proliferating uncontrollably.

This defiance stems from mutations in critical genes that regulate cell division, growth, and death. These mutated genes can be categorized into two main classes:

Oncogenes: These act like overenthusiastic conductors, constantly pushing the orchestra to play louder and faster, promoting uncontrolled cell division.

Tumor suppressor genes: Conversely, these function as the calming counterpoint, ensuring the orchestra plays at the appropriate tempo by regulating cell growth and initiating programmed cell death (apoptosis) when cells are damaged or no longer needed.

The unchecked growth of cancer cells disrupts the delicate balance of tissues, forming tumors. These tumors can be benign, meaning they remain localized and don't invade surrounding tissues. However, malignant tumors, the hallmark of cancer, possess an additional sinister ability: invasion and metastasis. Malignant cells develop the capacity to break away from the primary tumor, infiltrate healthy tissues, and establish secondary tumors throughout the body. This metastatic spread is the leading cause of death in cancer patients.

Tumors can be benign, meaning they do not spread to other parts of the body, or malignant, meaning they invade nearby tissues and can metastasize to distant sites.

The transformation of a normal cell into a cancerous one typically involves a series of genetic changes. These changes can be triggered by a variety of factors, including environmental exposures (such as tobacco smoke or radiation), inherited genetic mutations, and random errors that occur during cell division.

One of the most well-known tumor suppressor genes is TP53, which codes for the p53 protein. Often referred to as the "guardian of the genome," p53 plays a crucial role in preventing cancer by repairing damaged DNA or triggering cell death when the damage is too severe. Mutations in the TP53 gene are found in more than half of all human cancers, highlighting its critical role in maintaining cellular integrity.

In addition to genetic changes, cancer cells also exhibit several other characteristics that distinguish them from normal cells. These include the ability to sustain proliferative signaling, evade growth suppressors, resist cell death, enable replicative immortality, induce angiogenesis (the formation of new blood vessels), and activate invasion and metastasis.

These traits, collectively known as the "hallmarks of cancer," provide a framework for understanding the complex biology of cancer and the various strategies that cancer cells use to thrive.

One of the key challenges in cancer treatment is the heterogeneity of the disease. Even within a single tumor, there can be a diverse population of cells with different genetic and phenotypic characteristics. This heterogeneity can make it difficult to develop effective treatments, as different subpopulations of cancer cells may respond differently to therapy. Moreover, cancer cells are highly adaptable and can develop resistance to treatment over time, further complicating the management of the disease.

Despite these challenges, significant progress has been made in our understanding of cancer biology over the past few decades. Advances in genomics, molecular biology, and biotechnology have provided new insights into the mechanisms underlying cancer development and progression. These insights have paved the way for the development of targeted therapies, which aim to specifically inhibit the molecular pathways that drive cancer growth.

For example, the discovery of the role of the HER2 gene in breast cancer led to the development of trastuzumab (Herceptin), a monoclonal antibody that targets the HER2 protein and inhibits the growth of HER2positive breast cancer cells. Similarly, the identification of the BCRABL fusion protein in chronic myeloid leukemia (CML) resulted in the development of imatinib (Gleevec), a targeted therapy that specifically inhibits the activity of this protein and has dramatically improved outcomes for patients with CML.

In addition to targeted therapies, immunotherapy has emerged as a promising approach to cancer treatment. Immunotherapy harnesses the power of the body's immune system to recognize and attack cancer cells. One of the most successful examples of immunotherapy is the use of immune checkpoint inhibitors, which block proteins that prevent the immune system from attacking cancer cells. By releasing these "brakes" on the immune system, checkpoint inhibitors can help to unleash a powerful antitumor response.

Another important area of research in cancer biology is the tumor microenvironment. The tumor microenvironment refers to the surrounding cells, molecules, and blood vessels that support and interact with cancer cells.

This microenvironment plays a crucial role in cancer progression, as it provides essential nutrients and growth factors, protects cancer cells from the immune system, and facilitates invasion and metastasis. Understanding the interactions between cancer cells and their microenvironment is critical for developing new therapeutic strategies.

One of the most intriguing aspects of cancer biology is the concept of cancer stem cells. Cancer stem cells are a small subpopulation of cells within a tumor that possess the ability to self-renew and give rise to new cancer cells. These cells are thought to be responsible for tumor initiation, maintenance, and recurrence, and they are often more resistant to conventional therapies than other cancer cells. Targeting cancer stem cells represents a promising strategy for eradicating tumors and preventing relapse.

Facing Cancer: The Emotional and Physical Impact

"Hope is the physician of each misery." – Irish Proverb

You've heard the diagnosis. The room felt like it was closing in, the doctor's words echoing in your mind: cancer. It's a word that throws everything into a chaotic spin, leaving you reeling with a cocktail of emotions – fear, anger, confusion, and perhaps even a strange sense of disbelief. You're not alone in this emotional rollercoaster. Millions of people around the world face cancer every year, and the initial shock is a universal experience.

See yourself standing on a mountain peak, the world spread out majestically before you. Suddenly, the ground beneath your feet crumbles, and you're plummeting into a seemingly bottomless abyss. From the moment the word 'cancer' is uttered, your world changes. It's not just a physical battle; it's an emotional rollercoaster that impacts every aspect of your life. The initial shock can leave you feeling numb, disbelief mixing with fear. "Why me?" "Why me?" "What did I do wrong?" These are the questions that haunt you when you confront the truth of the situation. The answers, often elusive, may never come, but the feelings are all too real.

The unknown looms large, filled with questions about treatment, prognosis, and the future. You might worry about the impact on your loved ones, your career, and your very sense of self.

Anger, too, is a frequent visitor. It might be directed at the unfair hand you've been dealt, at the perceived injustice of a healthy body betraying you. You might feel angry at the world, at fate, or even at yourself. These emotions are valid, and bottling them up won't help. Find a safe space to express your anger, whether it's through journaling, talking to a therapist, or confiding in a trusted friend or family member.

The emotional toll doesn't exist in a vacuum. Cancer can wreak havoc on your physical wellbeing as well. Fatigue becomes a constant companion, sapping your energy and leaving you feeling drained. The very thought of even the simplest tasks can feel insurmountable. Treatment itself can come with a barrage of side effects, from nausea and vomiting to hair loss and mouth sores. These physical challenges can exacerbate the emotional turmoil, creating a vicious cycle that can be incredibly difficult to manage.

The first days after the diagnosis are a blur. You are thrust into a world of medical jargon and appointments. There's the biopsy, the scans, the consultations with oncologists.

Each visit to the hospital is a reminder of your new reality. You watch as doctors and nurses' bustle about, their faces kind but focused. You sit in waiting rooms filled with others who share your plight, some with haunted eyes, and others with a resolute determination that gives you a glimmer of hope.

You find yourself living in a world of "before" and "after." Before cancer, life was predictable, filled with routine and normalcy. After cancer, every day is a challenge, filled with appointments, treatments, and the constant presence of this uninvited guest in your life. It's exhausting, physically and emotionally. You're tired in a way you've never been before, a bone deep weariness that sleep can't seem to cure.

Treatment begins, and with it comes a new set of challenges. Chemotherapy, radiation, surgery – each has its own set of side effects. Your body, once strong and capable, now feels foreign. There's the nausea, the hair loss, the weight fluctuations. Your skin changes, your energy levels plummet. It's as if your body is no longer your own, hijacked by both the disease and the treatment meant to save you.

The emotional impact of cancer extends beyond you; it affects everyone around you. Your family and friends are thrown into their own turmoil.

They struggle to find the right words, to be strong for you when inside they're falling apart. You see the worry in their eyes, the forced smiles, the whispered conversations they think you don't hear. Cancer doesn't just affect you; it affects everyone you love.

There are times when you feel isolated, even in a room full of people. It's a loneliness that's hard to describe, a sense that no one truly understands what you're going through. You are not alone in this. Each of us has a story, a life that was unfolding in its unique pattern before cancer appeared uninvited. Perhaps you were planning a wedding, about to start a new job, or looking forward to retirement. Cancer doesn't discriminate; it can touch anyone, at any time. But it's not just an individual battle; it's a shared struggle that brings us together in a community bound by resilience and hope.

As you navigate the complexities of cancer, remember that your stories are powerful. They are narratives of struggle, yes, but also of hope and survival. They are reminders that, even in the darkest of times, the human spirit is capable of extraordinary resilience.

Your journey with cancer is not just a path marked by medical milestones; it's a testament to the enduring power of hope and the unyielding strength that lies within each of you.

Again, remember you are not alone in this fight. There is a vast community of people, both medical professionals and fellow patients, standing beside you. There will be good days and bad days, but with the right support system, a positive mindset, and a focus on self-care, you can emerge from this experience stronger and more empowered than ever before.

As you continue to face cancer, know that your experiences resonate with a chorus of others who walk this path alongside you. Together, we will face the storm, and together, we will seek the calm that follows. This is not just a chapter in a book; it's a chapter in your life, one that speaks of pain and healing, of battles and victories. And through it all, it's a chapter that continues to be written with courage, with love, and with an unwavering hope that endures.

Why Food Matters: Separating Fact from Fiction

You are what you eat, is an adage that takes on profound new meaning when facing a cancer diagnosis. In the whirlwind of emotions and medical appointments, the role of food can easily get relegated to the background. But here's the truth – food is not just sustenance; it's a powerful ally in your fight against cancer. When you're fighting cancer, every bite counts. The right nutrition can help your body stay strong during treatment, aid in recovery, and even improve your overall quality of life.

Imagine your body as a battlefield. Cancer cells are the enemy, relentlessly multiplying and wreaking havoc. But within you lies a vast network of warriors – your immune system. By strategically choosing the right foods, you can empower these warriors, giving them the ammunition they need to fight effectively.

The internet is a vast, and sometimes confusing, landscape when it comes to cancer and diet. Countless articles and "miracle cures" bombard you with conflicting information. It's easy to feel overwhelmed and unsure where to turn. Let's separate fact from fiction and explore the science behind why food truly matters in your recovery from cancer.

Understanding the Basics

Cancer treatments, while lifesaving, take a toll on the body. They can weaken the immune system, cause weight loss, fatigue, and other side effects that make the fight even harder. This is where nutrition steps in as a critical player. Proper nutrition provides the body with the essential vitamins, minerals, and nutrients it needs to repair tissues, maintain muscle mass, and boost the immune system.

However, it's important to note that no single diet or food can cure cancer. Instead, a balanced and varied diet can support conventional treatments and improve outcomes. Think of it as giving your body the tools it needs to fight back more effectively.

Myth 1: There's a "Cancer Fighting" Diet

The internet might lead you to believe there's a magic bullet diet that can cure cancer. Unfortunately, it's not that simple. Cancer is a complex disease, and there's no single dietary approach that guarantees a cure.

However, a well-planned, personalized diet rich in essential nutrients can significantly impact your journey.

For instance, some patients may experience loss of appetite or difficulty eating certain foods due to treatment side effects. In such cases, it's important to focus on nutrient dense foods that are easier to consume, like smoothies, soups, and pureed meals. The goal is to ensure adequate calorie and protein intake to prevent malnutrition and muscle loss. Think of it as a multipronged attack on the battlefield.

Fact: Food Can Boost Your Immune System

Your immune system is your body's defense mechanism, constantly on the lookout for invaders like bacteria, viruses, and even cancer cells. Nutrient rich foods can enhance your immune function, making it more effective in identifying and attacking cancer cells.

Foods high in antioxidants, such as berries, nuts, and green leafy vegetables, are particularly beneficial. Antioxidants help neutralize free radicals, unstable molecules that can damage cells and lead to cancer. Vitamin C (found in citrus fruits and bell peppers), vitamin E (found in nuts and seeds), and selenium (found in Brazil nuts and seafood) are powerful antioxidants that play a crucial role in immune health.

- **Managing Side Effects**: Cancer treatments, while crucial, can leave you feeling depleted. Proper nutrition can help manage common side effects like fatigue, nausea, and mouth sores, improving your overall wellbeing and treatment tolerance. For example, ginger can help alleviate nausea, while protein rich foods can combat fatigue.

- **Boosting Immunity**: A robust immune system is your body's natural defense system. Certain dietary components like vitamins A, C, and D, along with zinc and antioxidants, can enhance immune cell function, helping your body recognize and eliminate cancer cells more effectively.

- **Promoting Healing and Repair**: Cancer treatments can damage healthy tissues. Consuming a diet rich in essential nutrients like protein, vitamins, and minerals provides the building blocks necessary for repair and regeneration.

Myth 2: You Should Avoid All Sugar

The idea that sugar "feeds" cancer is a persistent myth that causes unnecessary anxiety. While it's true that all cells, including cancer cells, use glucose for energy, eliminating all sugar from your diet isn't practical or beneficial.

Instead, focus on reducing added sugars and refined carbohydrates, which can lead to weight gain and other health issues. Natural sugars found in fruits, vegetables, and whole grains are part of a healthy, balanced diet and provide essential nutrients and fiber.

Fact: Limiting Processed Foods is Key

Processed foods are often loaded with added sugar, unhealthy fats, and sodium. These can contribute to inflammation, a risk factor for cancer progression. Limiting processed foods and sugary drinks allows your body to focus its energy on healing and fighting cancer, not on processing unhealthy ingredients.

Myth 3: All Fats Are Bad

Not all fats are created equal. While it's wise to limit saturated and Trans fats found in processed foods and red meat, healthy fats are an important part of a balanced diet. Omega3 fatty acids, in particular, have anti-inflammatory properties and can support heart health and brain function.

Good sources of healthy fats include fatty fish (like salmon and mackerel), flaxseeds, chia seeds, walnuts, and olive oil. These fats can also help maintain energy levels and support the absorption of fat-soluble vitamins (A, D, E, and K).

Fact: Protein is Crucial for Healing and Strength

Protein is required to maintain muscular mass, heal tissues, and promote immunological function. During cancer treatment, your body needs more protein than usual to recover from the stress of treatments and rebuild strength.

Lean meats, poultry, fish, eggs, dairy products, beans, and legumes are excellent sources of protein. If eating solid foods is challenging, consider protein rich snacks like Greek yogurt, cottage cheese, or protein shakes. Including a source of protein with each meal and snack can help ensure you're meeting your body's needs.

Myth 4: Supplements Can Replace a Balanced Diet

While supplements can be helpful for filling nutritional gaps, they shouldn't replace a balanced diet. Whole foods provide a complex array of nutrients that work together in ways that supplements alone can't replicate.

Before taking any supplements, it's essential to consult with your healthcare team. Some supplements can interact with cancer treatments or other medications, potentially causing harm. Your doctor or dietitian can help determine if supplements are necessary and recommend safe options.

Fact: Hydration is Key

Staying hydrated is crucial, especially during cancer treatment. Dehydration can exacerbate treatment side effects like fatigue and nausea and can also lead to kidney problems if not addressed.

Water is the best choice for staying hydrated, but if plain water is unappealing, try flavored water, herbal teas, or broths. Foods with high water content, like cucumbers, watermelon, and oranges, can also contribute to your fluid intake. Aim to drink small amounts regularly throughout the day to maintain hydration.

Myth 5: You Need Restrictive Diets

Feeling overwhelmed by a mountain of restrictions is counterproductive. The goal is to create a sustainable, enjoyable eating pattern that nourishes your body. Focus on including a variety of nutrient rich foods from all food groups, rather than what you can't have.

Fact: Personalization is Key

There's no one size fits all approach to dietary changes. Your individual needs, preferences, and treatment plan should guide your dietary choices.

Working with a registered dietitian experienced in oncology can help you create a personalized plan that empowers you to take control of your health journey.

The Emotional Connection to Food

Food isn't just about nutrients and calories; it's also about comfort, tradition, and connection. During a time of illness, the emotional aspect of eating can be incredibly powerful.

Cooking and sharing meals with loved ones can provide a sense of normalcy and joy. It can also be a way to involve family and friends in your recovery journey. Simple acts like preparing a favorite dish or enjoying a meal together can create moments of happiness and support.

Embracing a New Reality

For many cancer patients, adjusting to new dietary needs can feel overwhelming. It's a shift in routine, and it can be challenging to stay motivated when you're feeling unwell. But remember, every positive change, no matter how small, can make a difference.

Begin by creating reasonable goals. Continue to incorporate more nutrient dense foods into your diet gradually. Celebrate little achievements, such as attempting a new healthy dish or consuming an entire meal despite side effects.

Don't be hesitant to seek assistance. A licensed dietician who specializes in cancer nutrition can offer individualized advice and assistance. They can help you navigate dietary changes, manage treatment side effects, and ensure you're getting the nutrients you need.

Food is more than simply nourishment; it is a kind of self-care. It's a way to take control of your health in a situation that often feels uncontrollable. It's a means to connect with loved ones, find comfort, and enjoy moments of pleasure even in difficult times.

Every meal you take is a step toward recovery. Embrace the power of nutrition, and let it be a source of strength and hope as you navigate your journey with cancer. Remember, you have the power to make choices that support your recovery and enhance your quality of life.

In the end, it's about more than just surviving – it's about thriving. It's about finding joy in the everyday moments, discovering new strengths, and embracing the future with hope. And through it all, let food be one of the many tools that help you on your path to recovery.

Chapter 2: Truth about Food as Medicine

"Let food be thy medicine and medicine be thy food." Attributed to Hippocrates, the father of modern medicine, this adage has found its way into numerous health promotion programs, championing the idea of "food as medicine." However, you may have encountered opposing viewpoints asserting, "No, food isn't medicine. It's food." Those online articles do not deny the significant role nutrition plays in health but challenge the often oversimplified interpretation of the "food as medicine" message.

A key issue arises when the notion of "food as medicine" is misunderstood to imply that proper diet alone can prevent all health issues, including cancer, or that dietary changes can cure cancer without medical intervention. This dangerous misinterpretation has led some to abandon essential medical treatments in favor of unproven dietary regimens, fueled by misinformation from social media and other unverified sources. It is vital to recognize that while healthy eating is crucial for cancer prevention and recovery, it does not replace the need for medical treatment.

Research strongly supports that healthy eating habits can lower the risk of cancer, heart disease, and diabetes. Adopting a healthy lifestyle, which includes a balanced diet, avoiding tobacco, limiting alcohol, and maintaining regular physical activity, can prevent about 42% of cancers. However, healthy eating alone is not a cure all. It is part of a comprehensive approach to reducing cancer risk and promoting overall health but does not guarantee immunity from disease.

Nutrition science has moved beyond the focus on individual nutrients or compounds. No single food can provide all the protective benefits necessary for cancer prevention. Instead, it is the pattern of healthy eating that offers the best protection. A varied diet rich in vitamins, minerals, phytochemicals, and dietary fiber works synergistically to reduce cancer risk and support general health.

Viewing food as medicine should not reduce it to a series of isolated, pharmaceutical like choices. This reductionist approach ignores the complexity of how nutrients work within the body.

Laboratory studies might show that a particular nutrient can switch off cancer related genes or enhance antioxidant defenses, but this does not mean that consuming foods containing that nutrient will have the same effect in the human body. The pathways through which nutrients operate are intricate and interdependent, as evidenced by various entries in the American Institute for Cancer Research's (AICR) Food Facts Library.

Moreover, reducing food purely to a medicinal function overlooks its broader context in our lives. Food is a vital part of cultural traditions, social connections, and personal pleasure. Limiting its role to merely a medicinal function diminishes its potential to enhance quality of life and emotional wellbeing.

At an AICR Lifestyle and Cancer Symposium, Dr. Dariush Mozaffarian emphasized that 80% of U.S. healthcare dollars are spent on chronic diseases, many of which are at least partially preventable through dietary choices. Evidence robustly supports that healthy eating habits can significantly reduce the burden of cancer and other chronic diseases.

Instead of focusing on individual foods as cures, we should prioritize long-term eating habits. This shift in perspective highlights that no single food offers complete protection.

Perhaps a more accurate phrase would be "diet as medicine," though this too can be misleading if people think of "diet" as a temporary fix. Instead, consider the concept of **"Healthy eating habits as medicine."** Sustainable eating patterns are where true health protection lies.

Healthy eating is a component of, not a replacement for, healthcare. Sometimes, healthy eating and an overall healthy lifestyle can prevent disease development. Other times, they help manage early warning signs or risk factors like inflammation or high blood pressure. When medical treatment is needed, it complements, rather than negates, the benefits of healthy eating. Together, they form a robust defense against illness.

Dr. Mozaffarian also emphasized that eating habits affect health through both beneficial and harmful foods. Consuming too little healthy food—such as whole grains, vegetables, and fruits—can increase cancer risk more than eating too much unhealthy food. Diets high in red and processed meats and sugar sweetened beverages also increase cancer risk. Sugar sweetened beverages, in particular, promote weight gain, which raises the risk of at least 12 different kinds of cancer. Thus, avoiding unintended weight gain is a crucial part of cancer risk reduction.

Healthy eating habits should not be conflated with any specific diet or eating pattern. The AICR Recommendations provide a blueprint for building healthy eating habits that fit individual and cultural preferences, emphasizing plant based foods. While some may choose to eat only plant based foods, the Recommendations simply call for plant focused eating habits.

Relying solely on plant based diets as the key to health can overlook crucial evidence. Research shows that even a plant based diet can be healthy or unhealthy depending on the quality of plant foods included. Presentations at the AICR Symposium highlighted that including more health promoting plant foods (like whole grains and vegetables) and fewer unhealthy plant foods leads to better outcomes for those living with and beyond cancer.

Even as we discuss food as medicine, the bigger picture is "lifestyle as medicine." Research shows that the best health outcomes are achieved when healthy eating is part of an overall healthy lifestyle. This includes regular physical activity, avoiding tobacco, and limiting or avoiding alcohol, as emphasized in the AICR Cancer Prevention Recommendations.

Implementing these Recommendations as a comprehensive package provides the greatest benefit. However, it's not an all-or-nothing approach. Each step toward healthier eating and lifestyle habits is a step toward better health.

Understanding the controversy over "food as medicine" shows that the disagreement lies in the overextension of the concept beyond what research supports. As part of an overall healthy eating pattern and lifestyle, the food you eat can help reduce cancer risk, support recovery, and be a delicious, enjoyable part of life.

When adopting new eating habits, especially those involving unfamiliar foods, it's important to learn how to prepare them in ways that fit your personal, family, and cultural preferences.

Food can indeed be medicine, but it requires a balanced, holistic approach to make it effective. By focusing on the quality and variety of your diet, you can harness the power of food to support your health and recovery. This approach, combined with appropriate medical care, provides the best chance for successful cancer prevention and treatment.

The journey of incorporating food as medicine is not just about combating cancer but also about enhancing overall wellbeing. It's about finding joy in the process, understanding the impact of your choices, and embracing a new perspective on eating. Each meal becomes a powerful step towards health, resilience, and recovery.

As cancer patients, it is essential to understand that while food is a powerful ally, it works best in conjunction with medical treatments. The synergy between a balanced diet and medical care can significantly improve outcomes, enhance quality of life, and support long-term health.

So, as you move forward, remember that your plate is a powerful tool in your fight against cancer. Embrace the diversity of nutritious foods, enjoy the flavors and textures, and let each meal be a testament to your strength and commitment to health.

Shifting Your Perspective on Eating

The food you eat can be either the safest and most powerful form of medicine or the slowest form of poison. This powerful statement by Ann Wigmore underscores the profound impact of dietary choices on health, particularly for cancer patients.

Malnutrition rates among cancer patients exceed 85%, with lung cancer, Glycemic Index (GI), and advanced stage malignancies bearing the most significant impact. Malnourished individuals tend to have worse reactions to chemotherapy, shorter survival rates, longer hospital admissions, and lower quality of life.

One promising intervention is Home Delivered Medically Tailored Meals (HDMTM), which are nutritionist prescribed meals tailored to patients' symptoms, comorbidities, and health needs. Preliminary data from 211 cancer patients showed that with HDMTM, 87% ate more than half of the meals, 91% lived more independently, 89% ate more nutritiously, and 70% had less fatigue. These meals could be a strategy to reduce financial toxicity and healthcare utilization while improving quality of life for cancer patients, though more primary data is needed to evaluate their efficacy.

Cancer is an aggressive disease often requiring aggressive treatment. The medical and scientific community is continually working to make cancer more manageable, akin to chronic diseases such as diabetes or heart disease. Oncology is evolving with novel methods for diagnosing and treating cancer.

Nutrition plays a crucial role in preventing cancer, supporting patients throughout treatment, and preventing recurrence in cancer survivors.

Nutritional oncology is a new field that combines precision nutrition and precision oncology to improve cancer prevention, treatment, and survival. According to Dr. David Heber, founding director of the UCLA Center for Human Nutrition, although research on the relationship between nutrition and cancer dates back far longer, it is only in the last 50 years that scientific data has revealed the numerous roles nutrition plays in cancer treatment.

In the 1920s, physicians believed that simply feeding the patient would cure cancer. However, as medicine advanced into the 1970s and 1980s, it became clear that nutritional support could aid patients alongside chemotherapy, surgery, or radiation. Recent research suggests that nutritional strategies effective for cancer prevention may also help prevent relapse after cancer treatment.

Recommending the same diet for every cancer patient is impractical due to the many variables involved, such as calorie expenditure, protein needs, and food allergies. The type and stage of cancer also matter when it comes to nutrition.

Nonetheless, certain nutrients should be part of the diet to ensure proper nourishment. Adequate protein and colorful fruits and vegetables, which carry antioxidants and fiber, help support the immune system and gastrointestinal tract.

A cancer patient's plate should be colorful, with various fruits and vegetables, each color representing beneficial antioxidant nutrients. Some natural foods that may help fight cancer include:

- **Broccoli**: Contains sulforaphane, which flushes out cancer causing chemicals.
- **Tomatoes**: Rich in lycopene, linked to preventing prostate, breast, and lung cancer, and reducing gastric cancer risk.
- **Berries (strawberries, raspberries, blackberries)**: Contain ellagic acid, which helps prevent cancer cell growth and improves the efficacy of some cancer drugs.
- **Pomegranates**: Their anti-inflammatory properties target certain proteins and genes to suppress cancer growth.

Nutrition is just one part of the cancer fighting strategy. It should be used as a measure for cancer prevention or to help patients stay in remission after successful treatment. Diet alone cannot cure cancer. A nutritious diet should complement proper treatments in cancer patients.

A study in 1981 indicated that roughly 35% of all cancers were related to diet. The American Institute for Cancer Research suggests that 50% of the most common cancers can be prevented by eating well, exercising, not smoking, protecting your skin, and getting vaccinated. Diet and lifestyle significantly impact cancer because of the way the tumor interacts with the surrounding tissue and cells, known as the microenvironment.

Seventy percent of the immune system is located in the gastrointestinal tract, which contains the microbiome. The microbiome, a community of bacteria, viruses, fungi, and other microbial cells, drives metabolism and immune function. Dysfunction in the microbiome can lead to excessive inflammation, promoting cancer development.

The microbiome is influenced by diet, lifestyle, and vitamins and minerals intake. When you eat, undigested food is broken down by the microbiome, creating bioactive substances that circulate throughout the body. Enhancing immunity through diet changes has been proven in studies.

Dr. Heber referenced a study tracking people successfully treated for cancer who later developed a different form of cancer. The study found that lifestyle played a major role in the development of the second cancer. While a healthy lifestyle does not guarantee cancer cure, measures such as reducing sugar intake, cutting back on refined carbohydrates, limiting red meat, getting the right amount of protein, and increasing fruit and vegetable intake can limit cancer risk.

The same nutrition used to prevent cancer initially can also be useful for cancer survivors. The importance of diet extends beyond prevention and can significantly impact cancer treatment and survival. It's essential to shift your perspective on eating to view food not just as sustenance but as a powerful tool in your cancer treatment and overall health strategy.

The microbiome's influence on the immune system is significant. A diet that supports a healthy microbiome can enhance your body's ability to fight cancer.

Understanding the impact of your diet on your health can empower you to make informed choices that support your treatment and recovery. While the journey of incorporating food as medicine involves making dietary changes, it also includes finding joy in eating and appreciating the flavors and textures of nutritious foods. Each meal becomes an opportunity to support your health and recovery.

Shifting your perspective on eating means recognizing that what you consume daily can profoundly affect your health. It's about understanding that every meal is an opportunity to nourish your body, support your treatment, and enhance your wellbeing. By focusing on the quality and variety of your diet, you can use food as a powerful tool in your fight against cancer.

This holistic approach, combined with appropriate medical care, provides the best chance for successful cancer prevention and treatment. By following a balanced, nutritious diet, you can enhance your quality of life, support your immune system, and improve your chances of recovery.

The Science behind Food's Power to Heal

When Urvi Shah, MD, was diagnosed with Hodgkin lymphoma in 2016, she was in the midst of her first year as a hematology oncology fellow. Despite her medical training, she was inundated with advice about what she should and shouldn't eat. As a budding oncologist, she assumed she already knew the optimal diet. However, her diagnosis led her to a startling realization: the specifics of nutrition, particularly in the context of cancer, were largely absent from her medical education.

Dr. Shah's experience underscores a significant gap in medical training. "We don't really get taught any of this in medical school," she notes. Her personal journey illuminated the natural desire of patients to feel empowered and take an active role in their health, particularly through diet and nutrition.

Her diagnosis and subsequent exploration into nutrition revealed a surprising truth about oncological advice. Traditionally, oncologists encouraged patients to eat whatever they wanted, believing that the rigors of cancer treatment were challenging enough without dietary restrictions.

This approach made sense when chemotherapy, known for causing nausea and vomiting, was the primary treatment. However, advancements in cancer therapies have made treatments more tolerable, shifting the focus to other health issues like diabetes, obesity, cardiovascular disease, and kidney disease, which often complicate cancer treatment.

Given these evolving dynamics, it's become evident that nutrition should play a crucial role in treatment plans for cancer patients. Dr. Shah's curiosity led her to ask why oncology lagged behind other specialties like cardiology and endocrinology, which have long-established dietary guidelines to support their treatments.

Shifting Focus to Cancer Diets

After joining Memorial Sloan Kettering Cancer Center (MSK) as a faculty member, Dr. Shah initially planned to focus on immunotherapy research. However, her personal battle with cancer redirected her interests towards diet and nutrition. In 2019, she proposed a pilot study on diet to her Service Chief, which quickly evolved into her primary research focus.

Her background and experience as a cancer patient fueled her dedication to formulating dietary guidelines for hematological malignancies, such as leukemia, lymphoma, and multiple myeloma. One pivotal question she sought to answer was whether diet could prevent conditions like monoclonal gammopathy of undetermined significance (MGUS) or smoldering myeloma from developing into multiple myeloma.

Investigating Diet's Impact on Cancer Progression

Dr. Shah embarked on her first study, a small clinical trial involving 20 participants with precursor conditions that could progress to cancer. Multiple myeloma, a cancer of plasma cells, often arises from MGUS or smoldering myeloma. Research indicates that individuals with these conditions who have an elevated body mass index (BMI) are twice as likely to develop multiple myeloma compared to those with a normal BMI.

This finding prompted Dr. Shah to conduct a study aimed at helping patients with an elevated BMI lose weight using healthy plant based foods. She partnered with Plantable, a company providing nutritional coaching and chef prepared, plant based meals.

Participants were allowed to consume whatever they liked, provided it was plant based, including fruits, vegetables, nuts, seeds, whole grains, and legumes. The high fiber content of these foods helps individuals feel full faster, potentially reducing overall calorie intake while providing high nutrient density.

A Patient's Journey: Will Wright

Will Wright's health struggles began in 2010 when he fainted after climbing three flights of stairs. Subsequent tests revealed he had both prostate cancer and kidney cancer. Despite surgical interventions, his anemia persisted. In 2016, MSK oncologist Sham Mailankody, MD, diagnosed him with MGUS, a condition that can progress to multiple myeloma but can often be managed to allow patients to live with it rather than succumb to it.

In mid-2019, Will began seeing Dr. Shah for MGUS monitoring. Overweight and a Type 2 diabetic for 30 years, he was an ideal candidate for Dr. Shah's pilot study on a vegan diet. Despite initial skepticism about abandoning his Southern cooking roots, Will embraced the plant based diet.

The transformation was remarkable. Within a month, Will no longer needed insulin and was no longer diabetic. His vision improved, his hair grew faster, and he lost 65 pounds. Surprisingly, he enjoyed his new vegan lifestyle and even learned to cook Thai food, which delighted his wife. Most importantly, his MGUS markers plateaued, suggesting that the progression of his condition might have been halted.

Broader Impacts and Success Stories

Will's case was not an isolated success. On average, participants in the initial trial lost about 8% of their body weight after 12 weeks. Many also experienced improved mental health, with one participant even discontinuing antidepressants.

These findings highlight the profound impact that dietary changes can have on health, particularly for cancer patients. The science behind food's power to heal is becoming increasingly clear. Whole, plant based foods provide essential nutrients and compounds that support the body's natural healing processes. By integrating these foods into your diet, you can potentially influence the progression of cancer and improve overall wellbeing.

Dr. Shah's research underscores the need for oncology to adopt comprehensive dietary guidelines similar to those in other medical fields. As you navigate your journey with cancer, consider the powerful role that nutrition can play in supporting your treatment and enhancing your quality of life. Embrace the science behind food's power to heal, and take an active role in your health through informed dietary choices.

Part 2: Building a Foundation for Optimal Nutrition

Chapter 3: Working with Your Medical Team

You've started this remarkable odyssey – a journey towards healing and reclaiming your health. This path may seem daunting at times, but remember you're not alone in this fight. Your medical team, a united force composed of your oncologist, registered dietitian (RD), and other healthcare professionals, stands firmly beside you. Building a strong, collaborative relationship with your team is paramount to achieving optimal nutrition alongside your medical treatment.

When navigating a cancer diagnosis and treatment, a collaborative approach with your medical team is essential. Optimizing your nutrition while undergoing medical treatment can significantly enhance your quality of life and improve treatment outcomes. Your oncologists are committed to working with you to develop a comprehensive, personalized plan that addresses your unique needs. Their goal is to support you every step of the way, ensuring you receive the best possible care and guidance.

Cancer treatment frequently includes a mix of surgery, chemotherapy, radiation, and targeted medicines.

Each of these treatments can have varying effects on your body and nutritional status. For instance, chemotherapy and radiation can cause side effects like nausea, vomiting, and loss of appetite, which can impact your ability to maintain adequate nutrition. By working closely with your medical team, including dietitians and nutritionists, you can develop strategies to manage these side effects and maintain your nutritional health.

The first step in this collaborative approach is **open communication**. It is crucial to share your dietary preferences, restrictions, and any symptoms you experience with your healthcare team. This information helps us tailor your nutritional plan to your specific needs and circumstances. Regularly updating us on how you feel allows us to adjust your treatment and nutritional recommendations as needed.

One of the key benefits of working with a multidisciplinary team is the integration of various expertise to support your health. Dietitians and nutritionists are invaluable members of your medical team. They can provide detailed nutritional assessments, identify potential deficiencies, and recommend dietary changes to enhance your wellbeing.

These professionals can help you navigate the complexities of maintaining a balanced diet during treatment, ensuring you receive adequate calories, protein, and essential nutrients.

A personalized nutrition plan is vital for managing cancer related symptoms and side effects. For example, if you are experiencing nausea or vomiting, a dietitian can suggest small, frequent meals that are easier to tolerate. They might recommend bland, low-fat foods and advise you to avoid strong odors that can exacerbate nausea. If you are struggling with a loss of appetite, they can suggest nutrient dense foods and strategies to stimulate your appetite, such as incorporating your favorite flavors and textures into meals.

Managing weight changes is another important aspect of your nutritional care. Weight loss can be a common issue during cancer treatment, leading to malnutrition and decreased strength. Conversely, some treatments can cause weight gain, which may lead to other health complications. Your medical team can help monitor your weight and adjust your diet to address these changes, ensuring you maintain a healthy weight throughout your treatment journey.

In addition to addressing immediate nutritional needs, your medical team will guide you in adopting long-term dietary habits that support your overall health and recovery. Emphasizing a plant based diet rich in fruits, vegetables, whole grains, and lean proteins can help boost your immune system and provide the energy you need for daily activities. Incorporating healthy fats, such as those found in nuts, seeds, and fatty fish, can also support your body's healing processes.

Hydration is another critical component of your nutritional plan. Cancer treatments can lead to dehydration, which can worsen symptoms like fatigue and nausea. Drinking plenty of fluids, such as water, herbal teas, and clear broths, can help keep you hydrated. Your dietitian can also recommend hydrating foods, like fruits and vegetables with high water content, to support your fluid intake.

Supplements may be necessary for some patients to address specific nutritional deficiencies. However, it is essential to discuss any supplements with your oncologist before taking them. Some supplements can interact with cancer treatments, potentially reducing their effectiveness or causing harmful side effects.

Your medical team will guide you on which supplements are safe and beneficial for your particular situation.

Your mental and emotional wellbeing is also an integral part of your overall health. Cancer treatment can be physically and emotionally draining, and maintaining a positive outlook can be challenging. Support groups, counseling, and mental health services are valuable resources that can provide emotional support and practical advice. Your healthcare team can help connect you with these resources to ensure you receive comprehensive care.

Engaging in regular physical activity, as tolerated, can also enhance your wellbeing. Exercise can help reduce fatigue, improve mood, and support overall physical health. Your oncologist and medical team can recommend appropriate exercises based on your treatment plan and physical condition. Activities like walking, gentle yoga, and stretching can be beneficial and can be adjusted according to your energy levels and abilities.

Being proactive in your care is crucial. Attend all scheduled appointments, and don't hesitate to ask questions or express concerns about your treatment or nutrition plan.

Keeping a journal of your symptoms, dietary intake, and any changes you notice can be a helpful tool for tracking your progress and communicating with your medical team.

Research is continually advancing our understanding of the role of nutrition in cancer care. Staying informed about new developments and discussing them with your healthcare team can help you make educated decisions about your diet and treatment. Your medical team is dedicated to providing you with the latest evidence based recommendations to support your health and recovery.

Building a strong support network is also essential. Family, friends, and caregivers can provide emotional support and practical assistance, such as preparing meals and helping with daily activities. Involving them in your care plan can help ensure you have the support you need to manage your treatment and maintain your nutritional health. Together, you can navigate the challenges of cancer treatment and work towards a healthier, brighter future.

Understanding Your Specific Needs and Diagnosis

Cancer is a catabolic inflammatory disease that often leads to significant weight loss, or in severe cases, cachexia. This undernourishment impairs your quality of life, reduces therapeutic response, and leads to a poor prognosis. Active and frequent nutritional screening and assessment using valid tools are crucial for fast and appropriate nutritional intervention. Based on these assessments, a suitable individualized nutritional intervention strategy can be established. Nutritional intervention typically begins with nutritional counseling, and a well-planned counseling session can improve treatment adherence and nutritional status.

Nutritional problems are common during cancer treatment. A prospective observational study reported that 51.1% of all cancer patients showed nutritional impairment, and 64% experienced weight loss six months after diagnosis. Weight loss, especially cachexia, is associated with reduced physical function, decreased quality of life, and poor prognosis. While Body mass index (BMI) is a traditional measure of nutritional status, recent studies have focused on sarcopenia.

Nutritional issues vary depending on the location and stage of cancer, making personalized nutritional support essential.

Cachexia in cancer patients is not simply due to malnutrition from anorexia. It is a complex condition involving reduced intake, metabolic dysfunction, and increased energy requirements. This process involves various inflammatory cytokines in cancer cells, alterations in protein and lipid metabolism, and an imbalance in muscle protein production and degradation.

Inflammation plays a significant role in cancer related nutritional metabolism. Increased inflammatory cytokines such as TNFα and interleukin6 (IL6) are critical in this process. TNFα, initially called cachectin, has been known to cause muscle mass loss in experimental models, and blocking TNFα in studies has shown some muscle preservation. IL6 is also crucial in cancer related cachexia. It is associated with muscle wasting through its effects on acute phase reactants and inflammatory pathways.

In cancer patients, protein production and degradation are regulated by catabolic stress through pathways like the ubiquitin proteasome pathway, autophagy, and transforming growth factor beta family ligands.

These processes lead to muscle wasting and decreased muscle strength, exacerbated by chemotherapy and related complications like microsites, which can directly induce muscle loss.

Cancer patients often experience impaired carbohydrate metabolism, with high rates of glycolysis in cancer cells and increased glucose production through gluconeogenesis in the liver. This results in high energy demands. Although insulin resistance is common, it is not always associated with weight loss. Lipid metabolism is also disrupted, with increased free fatty acids and glycerol from triglycerides promoting cachexia. Fat browning, where white adipose tissue converts to beige cells, further contributes to metabolic imbalance and energy expenditure through thermogenesis.

Maintaining weight is crucial for a better prognosis. Malnutrition is linked to longer hospital stays, higher infection rates, delayed wound healing, immune system deterioration, and increased cancer related mortality.

Sarcopenia, the loss of muscle mass, is a significant factor in poor prognosis, impacting chemotherapy toxicity, tumor progression, and survival rates.

The quality of life in cancer patients is significantly influenced by nutritional status. Weight loss and decreased appetite are closely related to poorer quality of life. However, improving nutritional status alone does not necessarily enhance quality of life. Tumor regression plays a crucial role in this improvement, indicating the complex relationship between cancer, malnutrition, and quality of life.

Assessing weight loss remains a simple and effective method to determine malnutrition. Body mass index (BMI), despite its limitations, continues to be an important tool. Studies show that unintentional weight loss and low Body mass index (BMI) are associated with poorer survival rates. However, excessive nutrition is not recommended, as it can worsen outcomes, particularly when muscle loss accompanies weight gain.

Nutritional screening tools, such as the Malnutrition Universal Screening Tool, Nutrition Risk Screening 2002, Mini Nutritional Assessment Short Form, and Malnutrition Screening Tool, are used to identify nutritional risk. These tools combine factors like BMI, weight change, food intake, and accompanying diseases to provide a comprehensive assessment.

Regular nutritional screening from the point of cancer diagnosis is recommended to prevent malnutrition and improve outcomes.

Once a nutritional risk is identified, a detailed assessment must follow. Comprehensive nutritional assessments involve evaluating medical history, dietary intake, physical activity, weight changes, and laboratory results. Tools like the patient generated subjective global assessment (PGSGA) are specifically designed for cancer patients, providing a reliable method to identify and classify nutritional states. This tool assesses various factors, including weight and dietary changes, gastrointestinal symptoms, and overall nutritional impact, guiding the start and follow-ups of nutritional interventions.

Understanding your specific needs and diagnosis is crucial in tailoring dietary plans for optimal results. Given the complex interplay between cancer, treatment, and nutrition, a personalized approach is necessary. This involves not only addressing the physical aspects of nutrition but also considering the emotional, psychological, and social dimensions of eating.

Your Doctor will begin by conducting a thorough assessment of your current health status, including your nutritional intake, weight, body composition, and symptoms. This information helps them to create a personalized plan that addresses your unique needs and preferences. Open communication is key. Share your dietary habits, preferences, and any difficulties you face with food. This dialogue allow them to design a plan that is not only nutritionally adequate but also enjoyable and sustainable.

Addressing preexisting conditions or comorbidities that affect your nutritional status is vital. Their multidisciplinary team will collaborate to ensure all aspects of your health are considered. Supplements may be recommended for specific deficiencies, but it is essential to approach supplementation with caution and under medical guidance.

The goal of your tailored dietary plan is to support your body during treatment, enhance your quality of life, and promote long-term health. By understanding your specific needs and working closely with your medical team, you can optimize your nutrition and improve your wellbeing. This collaborative approach ensures your dietary plan is effective, practical, and enjoyable, helping you navigate the challenges of cancer treatment with resilience and confidence.

Your journey is unique, and your dietary needs will evolve. Stay engaged with your medical team, keep an open mind, and be willing to make adjustments as needed. Together, you can create a nutritional plan that supports your health, enhances your treatment, and helps you achieve the best possible outcomes. Your commitment to understanding and meeting your specific needs is a vital part of your overall cancer care strategy, and they will always be available to support you every step of the way.

Chapter 4: Understanding Macronutrients and Micronutrients

Understanding the role of macronutrients and micronutrients is crucial for maintaining your overall health, supporting your immune system, and enhancing your treatment outcomes during cancer therapy. These essential components of your diet play significant roles in cellular structure, function, and physiological regulation, affecting everything from hormone levels to cellular signaling pathways. Proper nutrition can reduce the risk of developing cancer and improve your response to treatment.

Macronutrients are nutrients that your body requires in large amounts to function properly. They include carbohydrates, proteins, and fats. Each macronutrient serves a unique and vital role in your body, providing energy, building and repairing tissues, and supporting various physiological functions.

Carbohydrates are your body's primary source of energy. They are broken down into glucose, which fuels your brain, muscles, and other tissues.

It is essential to focus on complex carbohydrates, such as whole grains, fruits, vegetables, and legumes, which provide sustained energy and are rich in fiber, vitamins, and minerals. These foods help stabilize blood sugar levels and support digestive health, both of which are crucial during cancer treatment. Simple carbohydrates, like those found in sugary snacks and refined grains, should be limited as they can cause spikes in blood sugar and lack essential nutrients.

Proteins are the building blocks of your body. They are composed of amino acids, which are necessary for repairing tissues, supporting the immune system, and maintaining muscle mass. Ensuring adequate protein intake is particularly important for cancer patients, as treatments like chemotherapy and radiation can lead to muscle wasting and increased protein needs. Good sources of protein include lean meats, poultry, fish, dairy products, eggs, legumes, nuts, and seeds. In some cases, protein supplements may be recommended to meet your requirements.

Fats are essential for various bodily functions, including hormone production, brain function, and the absorption of fat soluble vitamins (A, D, E, and K). It is important to incorporate healthy fats into your diet, such as those found in avocados, nuts, seeds, olive oil, and fatty fish.

These foods not only provide essential nutrients but also help combat inflammation, which can be a concern for cancer patients. Limiting saturated and Trans fats, often found in processed foods, can further support your health and reduce the risk of inflammation related complications.

While macronutrients are needed in larger quantities, micronutrients, which include vitamins and minerals, are required in smaller amounts but are equally crucial for your health. They play a vital role in various biochemical processes, supporting immune function, energy production, and overall cellular health.

Vitamins are organic compounds necessary for normal growth and development. Vitamins are classified as either fat soluble or water-soluble. Fat-soluble vitamins (A, D, E, and K) are stored in the body's fatty tissues and liver, and can be accessed when needed. Water-soluble vitamins (B complex and C) are not stored in the body and need to be consumed regularly through your diet.

Vitamin A is necessary for normal eyesight, skin, and immunological function. It is found in foods like carrots, sweet potatoes, spinach, and liver. Vitamin D, often referred to as the "sunshine vitamin," is crucial for bone health and immune function.

It can be obtained from sunlight exposure, fatty fish, fortified dairy products, and supplements if necessary. Vitamin E acts as a powerful antioxidant, protecting cells from damage, and is found in nuts, seeds, and vegetable oils. Vitamin K is important for blood clotting and bone health, and can be found in leafy green vegetables, such as kale and spinach.

The Bcomplex vitamins, including B1 (thiamine), B2 (riboflavin), B3 (niacin), B6 (pyridoxine), B9 (folate), and B12 (cobalamin), play diverse roles in energy production, red blood cell formation, and neurological function. These vitamins are found in a variety of foods, including whole grains, meats, dairy products, leafy greens, and legumes. Vitamin C, another water-soluble vitamin, is essential for collagen production, wound healing, and immune function. It is abundant in citrus fruits, strawberries, bell peppers, and broccoli.

Minerals are inorganic elements critical for various bodily functions, including bone health, fluid balance, and muscle contraction. Key minerals include calcium, iron, magnesium, potassium, and zinc.

Calcium is essential for both bone health and muscular function. It is present in dairy products, leafy green vegetables, and fortified meals.

Iron is essential for oxygen transfer in the blood and energy generation. It can be obtained from red meat, poultry, fish, legumes, and fortified cereals. Magnesium plays a role in over 300 biochemical reactions in the body, including muscle and nerve function, and is found in nuts, seeds, whole grains, and green leafy vegetables. Potassium is essential for maintaining fluid balance, nerve function, and muscle contractions, and is abundant in fruits, vegetables, and legumes. Zinc supports immune function, wound healing, and DNA synthesis, and is found in meat, shellfish, legumes, and seeds.

During cancer treatment, your body's demand for certain vitamins and minerals may increase due to the stress of the disease and the effects of treatment. For instance, chemotherapy can lead to increased oxidative stress, necessitating higher antioxidant intake to protect cells from damage.

Additionally, treatments can cause side effects like nausea, vomiting, and diarrhea, which can deplete your body's nutrient stores.

To ensure you are meeting your nutritional needs, regular monitoring and assessment are essential.

This involves blood tests to check for deficiencies, as well as consultations with your healthcare team to adjust your dietary plan as needed. In some cases, supplementation may be necessary to address specific deficiencies, but it is crucial to do so under the guidance of your medical team to avoid potential interactions with cancer treatments.

Understanding the balance of macronutrients and micronutrients in your diet is not just about meeting basic nutritional needs; it is about optimizing your body's ability to fight cancer, support recovery, and maintain overall health. A well rounded diet that includes a variety of nutrient dense foods can help you manage treatment side effects, boost your immune system, and improve your quality of life.

Demystifying Macronutrients: Protein, Carbs, and Fat

In the complex world of nutrition, macronutrients play a pivotal role in shaping our overall health and wellbeing. Carbohydrates, proteins, and fats are the basic components of our food, supplying energy for biological operations and regulating vital processes. Understanding the power of these macronutrients is essential for making sound dietary decisions and living a healthy lifestyle. Here, I move into the intricacies of carbohydrates, proteins, and fats, unraveling the mysteries behind their functions and highlighting their significance in our daily lives.

Carbohydrates 101

Carbohydrates are your body's preferred energy source, providing fuel for various physiological activities. When consumed, carbohydrates turn into glucose (also known as blood sugar) and play a key role in functions such as digestion, gut health, and cognitive function. Carbohydrates are classified as either simple or complex. Simple carbohydrates are composed of one (monosaccharide) or two (disaccharide) sugar units. They taste sweet and are broken down quickly by your body. For instance, when you reach for a doughnut to get through the afternoon slump and experience a quick spike of energy followed by a crash, that's simple carbs at work.

Simple carbohydrates, found in foods like fruits and honey, are quickly converted into glucose, offering a rapid energy boost. Complex carbs, found in meals such as whole grains and vegetables, provide continuous energy since they take longer to digest. Whole, unprocessed carbohydrates are crucial for maintaining a consistent source of energy and promoting overall health.

Simple carbohydrates include baked products, soda, and refined sugar, all of which should be taken in moderation. However, many healthful foods, such as milk and fruit, include simple carbohydrates.

Whole grains, starchy vegetables, potatoes, oats, rice, and pulses are excellent sources of complex carbohydrates. Dietary guidelines recommend aiming to get 45%-65% of your total daily calories from carbs. Emphasizing these healthier carbohydrate choices can help maintain your energy levels and support your body's essential functions, especially during cancer treatment.

Protein 101

Proteins are the building blocks of your body, responsible for repairing and building tissues, synthesizing enzymes and hormones, and supporting the immune system. Comprising amino acids, proteins play a vital role in muscle development and repair. Consuming a variety of protein sources, such as lean meats, fish, eggs, dairy products, legumes, and nuts, ensures that your body receives all the essential amino acids it needs.

Adequate protein intake is particularly crucial for individuals undergoing cancer treatment, as it aids in muscle recovery and growth, which can be compromised due to muscle wasting from treatments like chemotherapy and radiation.

Proteins are composed of 20 amino acids, of which nine are considered essential, meaning your body needs them to function and cannot produce them on its own. Foods that contain all nine essential amino acids are called complete proteins and include fish, poultry, eggs, dairy products, beef, pork, and soy products such as tofu. Other protein sources include nuts and seeds, whole grains, veggies, and legumes.

The recommended daily allowance of protein is around 0.8 grams per kilogram of body weight (or 0.36 grams per pound). This amount can vary based on individual needs, particularly during periods of increased physical activity or stress, such as cancer treatment. Ensuring that you consume adequate protein can help support your immune system, maintain muscle mass, and improve overall treatment outcomes.

Fat 101

Contrary to the misconception that all fats are harmful, fats are essential for overall health. They serve as a concentrated source of energy, aid in the absorption of fat soluble vitamins (A, D, E, and K), and play a crucial role in brain health. Fats are made up of smaller molecules known as fatty acids, which serve important roles in your body such as producing energy, protecting cells, fighting inflammation, and delaying digestion, which allows you to feel fuller for longer and helps you avoid overeating.

There are two forms of fat: saturated and unsaturated. Saturated fats are normally solid at room temperature, whereas unsaturated fats are frequently liquid. Both types are essential for your health, but saturated fats can also raise your LDL (bad) cholesterol levels and should be consumed in moderation. Examples of foods high in saturated fat include milk, cheese, butter, and some meats like beef and pork.

Unsaturated fats have numerous health benefits and may help reduce the risk of heart disease, improve cholesterol levels, and promote overall good health.

Examples of monounsaturated fats include olive oil, avocados, nuts, and seeds, while polyunsaturated fats are found in fatty fish, soybeans, walnuts, chia seeds, and hemp seeds. Trans fats, which have no nutritional value and might be damaging to your health, should be avoided or ingested in moderation. These fats are found in fried foods, processed foods, and baked goods.

Experts recommend consuming no more than 30 grams of saturated fat per day for men and 20 grams for women. Your daily total fat intake should make up 20%-35% of your overall daily calories, with monounsaturated fats making up the majority of this intake. Additionally, fats are involved in hormone regulation, making them vital for various bodily functions, including reproductive health and mood regulation.

Achieving a balanced intake of carbohydrates, proteins, and fats is essential for optimal health and wellbeing. The right balance varies based on individual factors such as age, activity level, and overall health goals. A well rounded diet includes a variety of whole foods, incorporating ample fruits, vegetables, whole grains, lean proteins, and healthy fats.

Monitoring portion sizes and being aware of the body's signals of hunger and fullness can also help you maintain a healthy macronutrient intake.

Understanding the influence of macronutrients is essential for making informed dietary choices that promote health. Carbohydrates, proteins, and fats are indispensable components of your diet, each serving unique functions in the body. Embracing a balanced approach to nutrition, incorporating a variety of whole foods rich in these macronutrients, empowers you to fuel your bodies optimally. By demystifying the roles of carbohydrates, proteins, and fats, you can embark on a journey toward better health, vitality, and overall wellbeing.

Remember that your nutritional needs may change during cancer treatment. Regular monitoring and consultations with your healthcare team are essential to adjust your diet as needed.

The Essential Micronutrients: Vitamins, Minerals, and Antioxidants

Micronutrients are an essential category of nutrients that your body needs. They include vitamins and minerals, which can be divided into macro minerals, trace minerals, and water and fat soluble vitamins. An adequate intake of micronutrients often means aiming for a balanced diet.

Vitamins are necessary for energy production, immune function, blood clotting, and other vital processes. Meanwhile, minerals play crucial roles in growth, bone health, fluid balance, and numerous other functions. Understanding these micronutrients is essential for maintaining overall health, especially during cancer treatment.

What are micronutrients?

The phrase micronutrients refers to vitamins and minerals in general. Unlike macronutrients, which include proteins, fats, and carbohydrates, your body needs smaller amounts of micronutrients. That's why they're labeled "micro." Humans must obtain micronutrients from food since your body cannot produce most vitamins and minerals on its own, making those essential nutrients.

Vitamins are organic compounds made by plants and animals, which can be broken down by heat, acid, or air. Minerals, on the other hand, are inorganic and exist in soil or water, remaining unchanged by these elements. When you eat, you consume the vitamins that plants and animals have created or the minerals they have absorbed.

Each food has a different micronutrient content, so it's best to eat a variety of foods to get a sufficient amount of vitamins and minerals. An appropriate consumption of all micronutrients is required for good health, as each vitamin and mineral serves a distinct function in your body. They are essential for growth, immunological function, brain development, and a variety of other crucial processes. Certain micronutrients can also help prevent and treat diseases.

Types and functions of micronutrients

Vitamins and minerals are classified into four categories: water-soluble vitamins, fat-soluble vitamins, macro minerals, and trace minerals. Regardless of type, vitamins and minerals are absorbed similarly in your body and interact in many processes.

Water-soluble vitamins

Most vitamins dissolve in water and are so classified as water soluble. They're not easily stored in your body and get flushed out with urine when consumed in excess. While each water soluble vitamin has a unique role, their functions are related. For example, most B vitamins act as coenzymes that help trigger important chemical reactions necessary for energy production.

The water soluble vitamins have the following functions:

- **Vitamin B1 (thiamine)**: Helps convert nutrients into energy.

- **Vitamin B2 (riboflavin)**: Necessary for energy production, cell function, and fat metabolism.

- **Vitamin B3 (niacin):** Promotes the generation of energy from foods.

- **Vitamin B5 (pantothenic acid)** is necessary for fatty acid production.

- **Vitamin B6 (pyridoxine)**: Allows your body to release sugar from stored carbs for energy and produce red blood cells.

- **Vitamin B7 (Biotin)**: is involved in the metabolism of fatty acids, amino acids, and glucose.

- **Vitamin B9 (folate):** Required for normal cell division.

- **Vitamin B12 (cobalamin)** is required for the development of red blood cells as well as normal nerve and brain function.

- **Vitamin C (ascorbic acid)** is required for the production of neurotransmitters and collagen, the primary protein in your skin.

Water-soluble vitamins help to produce energy and perform other activities. Because these vitamins cannot be stored in the body, they must be obtained through diet. The sources and recommended dietary allowances (RDAs) or adequate intakes (AIs) of water soluble vitamins are:

Nutrients	Source	RDA or AI (adults > 19 years)
Vitamin B1 (thiamine)	Whole grain, meat, fish	1.1-1. 2 mg
Vitamin B2 (riboflavin)	Organ meat, eggs, milk	1.1-1.3 mg
Vitamin B3 (niacin)	Meat, salmon, leafy greens, beans	14-16 mg
Vitamin B5 (pantothenic acid)	Organ meats, mushroom, tuna, avocado	5 mg
Vitamin B6 (pyridoxine)	Fish, milk, carrot, potatoes	1.3-1.7 mg
Vitamin B7 (Biotin)	Eggs, almonds, spinach, sweet potatoes	30 mcg
Vitamin B9 (folate)	Beef, liver, Black-eye peas, spinach, asparagus	400 mcg

| Vitamin B12 (cobalamin) | Clams, fish, meat | 2.4 mcg |
| Vitamin C (ascorbic acid) | Citrus fruits, bell peppers, Brussels, sprouts | 75-90 mg |

Fat-soluble vitamins

Fat-soluble vitamins do not dissolve in water. They are most effectively absorbed when ingested with a source of fat. Following ingestion, fat-soluble vitamins are stored in your liver and fatty tissues for later use.

The names and functions of fat-soluble vitamins are:

- **Vitamin A**: Essential for maintaining healthy vision, skin, and immune function. Found in foods like carrots, sweet potatoes, spinach, and liver.

- **Vitamin D**: Crucial for bone health and immune function. It can be obtained from sunlight exposure, fatty fish, fortified dairy products, and supplements if necessary.

- **Vitamin E:** Acts as a powerful antioxidant, protecting cells from damage. Found in nuts, seeds, and vegetable oils.

- **Vitamin K:** Important for blood clotting and bone health. Found in leafy green vegetables, such as kale and spinach.

The sources and suggested intakes of fat-soluble vitamins are:

Nutrients	Source	RDA or AI (adults > 19 years)
Vitamin A	Retinol (liver, dairy, fish), carotenoids (sweet potatoes, carrots, spinach)	700-900 mcg
Vitamin D	Sunlight, fish oil, milk	15-20 mcg
Vitamin E	Sunflower seeds, wheat germ, almonds	15 mg
Vitamin K	Leafy greens, soybeans, pumpkin	90-120 mcg

Macro minerals

Macro minerals are required in bigger quantities than trace minerals to execute their unique functions in your body.

The macro minerals and some of their functions include:

- Calcium is necessary for the healthy formation and function of bones and teeth. Promotes muscular function and blood vessel contraction.

- Phosphorus is a component of bone and cell membrane structures.

- Magnesium: Helps regulate over 300 enzyme processes, including blood pressure.

- Sodium is an electrolyte that helps to balance fluids and maintain blood pressure.

- Chloride is commonly seen in conjunction with sodium. It promotes fluid equilibrium and is utilized to create digestive juices.

- Potassium is an electrolyte that helps cells maintain fluid balance and aids nerve transmission and muscle function.

- Sulfur is found in every living tissue, including the amino acids methionine and cysteine.

Sources and recommended macro mineral intakes are:

Nutrients	Source	RDA or AI (adults > 19 years)
Calcium	Milk product, leafy greens, broccoli	1000-1200 mg
Phosphorus	Salmond, yogurt, turkey	700 mg
Magnesium	Almonds, cashews, black beans	310-420 mg
Sodium	Salt, processed foods, canned soup	1500 mg
Chloride	Seaweed, salt, celery	1800-2300 mg
Potassium	Lentils, acorn squash, bananas	2600-3400 mg
Sulphur	Garlic, onions, Brussels sprouts, eggs, mineral water	Non established

Trace minerals

Trace minerals are required in lesser proportions than macro minerals but nevertheless play vital roles in the body.

The trace minerals and their roles include:

- **Iron:** Helps deliver oxygen to muscles and aids in the production of certain hormones.
- **Manganese** promotes glucose, amino acid, and cholesterol metabolism.
- **Copper** is required for connective tissue production as well as proper brain and nervous system function.
- **Zinc** is necessary for healthy development, immunological function, and wound healing.
- **Iodine:** Helps regulate thyroid function.
- **Fluoride** is required for the formation of bones and teeth.
- **Selenium** is essential for thyroid function, reproduction, and antioxidant defense.

The sources and suggested intakes of trace minerals are:

Nutrients	Source	RDA or AI (adults > 19 years)
Iron	Oysters, white beans, spinach	8-18 mg
Manganese	Pineapple, pecans, peanuts	1.8-2.3 mg
Copper	Liver, crabs, cashews	900 mcg
Zinc	Oysters, crab, chickpeas	8-11 mg
Iodine	Seaweed, cod, chickpeas	150 mcg
Fluoride	Fruits juice, water, crab	3-4 mg
Selenium	Brazil nuts, sardines, ham	55 mcg

Essential micronutrients include vitamins, minerals, and antioxidants.

Health Benefits of Micronutrients

All micronutrients are critical for the healthy functioning of your body. A balanced diet rich in vitamins and minerals is essential for good health and may even aid in illness prevention. This is because micronutrients are involved in almost every activity in your body. Furthermore, several vitamins and minerals can function as antioxidants.

Antioxidants may defend against cell damage, which has been linked to several disorders such as cancer, obesity, and cardiovascular disease.

For example, studies have linked an appropriate dietary intake of vitamins A and C to a decreased risk of some forms of cancer. Consuming enough iron and copper in your diet may help slow the course of Alzheimer's disease.

Certain minerals may also help prevent and treat illness. Low selenium levels in the blood have been related to an increased risk of heart disease. According to a previous assessment of observational data, increasing blood selenium concentrations by 50% reduced the incidence of heart disease by 24%. These studies demonstrate that ingesting enough amounts of all micronutrients, particularly those with antioxidant characteristics, has several health advantages.

However, it is uncertain if ingesting more than the recommended levels of specific micronutrients, whether through meals or supplements, provides extra advantages.

Micronutrient deficiencies and toxicities

Micronutrients require certain levels to complete their respective roles in the body. Excessive or insufficient vitamin or mineral intake might result in harmful side effects.

Deficiencies

Most healthy individuals can obtain enough micronutrients from a balanced diet, however there are several frequent nutritional shortages that affect specific groups. This includes:

- **Vitamin D:** Many Americans are vitamin D deficient, primarily owing to a lack of sun exposure.

- **Vitamin B12:** By avoiding animal products, vegans and vegetarians may develop a vitamin B12 deficiency. Elderly people are additionally at danger since their absorption rate decreases with age.

- **Vitamin A:** Women and children's diets in poor nations frequently lack enough vitamin A levels.

- **Iron** deficiency is frequent among preschool children, menstrual women, and vegetarians.

- **Calcium**: Approximately 22% of men and 10% of women over 50 do not get adequate calcium.

The indications, symptoms, and long term repercussions of these deficiencies vary depending on the vitamin, but they can be harmful to your body's healthy functioning and overall health.

Toxicities

Micronutrient toxicity is less prevalent than deficiency. They are particularly likely to develop with high doses of fat soluble vitamins A, D, E, and K, which can be stored in your liver and fatty tissues. They cannot be eliminated from your body like water soluble vitamins.

Micronutrient toxicity is most commonly caused by excessive supplementation, rather than dietary sources. The signs and symptoms of poisoning differ based on the nutrient. It is crucial to note that even if no overt poisoning symptoms appear, over ingestion of some minerals can be harmful.

Micronutrient supplements

The safest and most effective approach to receive enough vitamins and minerals appears to be through dietary sources. More study is needed to properly understand the long term consequences of toxicants and supplements. People who are at risk of certain vitamin deficiencies, on the other hand, may benefit from taking supplements as prescribed by a doctor. If you want to take micronutrient supplements, check for third party certified goods. Unless expressly instructed by a healthcare expert, avoid goods with "super" or "mega" doses of any vitamin.

Part 3: Supporting Your Body through Treatment

Chapter 5: Managing Treatment Side Effects with Food

"The body is a garden," Voltaire once remarked, "and it's our duty to cultivate it."

This sentiment holds particular weight for cancer patients navigating the often tumultuous terrain of treatment. In the journey through cancer treatment, patients often encounter a myriad of side effects that can affect their quality of life and overall wellbeing. Among these, the impact on nutrition and the ability to maintain a healthy diet is significant. The intersection of oncology and nutrition offers a unique opportunity to manage and mitigate these side effects, not just with medication, but with the very sustenance of life: food.

The concept of using food as a tool to manage the side effects of cancer treatment is rooted in the understanding that what we eat can influence our body's reactions. Cancer treatments, while targeting malignant cells, can inadvertently affect normal cells and physiological processes, leading to side effects that range from mild to debilitating.

These can include nausea, vomiting, altered taste sensations, loss of appetite, and gastrointestinal disturbances, among others. The role of optimal nutrition becomes paramount in this context, serving as a complementary strategy to traditional medical interventions.

One of the primary concerns during cancer treatment is the management of gastrointestinal side effects such as nausea and vomiting. These symptoms can lead to a decreased intake of food and fluids, resulting in weight loss and malnutrition. To combat this, small, frequent meals that are easy on the stomach and rich in nutrients can be beneficial. Foods like ginger, peppermint, and crackers are often recommended for their anti-nausea properties. Additionally, staying hydrated with small sips of water or electrolyte rich beverages throughout the day can help prevent dehydration.

Another common side effect is a change in taste or smell, which can make food less appealing and lead to a reduced desire to eat. Experimenting with different flavors, textures, and temperatures can help in finding foods that are more palatable. Adding herbs, spices, and sauces can enhance the taste of food and stimulate appetite. For those experiencing a metallic taste, using plastic utensils and avoiding canned foods can be helpful.

Loss of appetite is also a challenge for many cancer patients. High calorie, nutrient dense foods can provide the energy and nutrients needed without requiring large portions. Smoothies, shakes, and soups can be packed with protein, healthy fats, and vitamins, making them an excellent choice for those struggling to eat solid foods.

For patients dealing with constipation or diarrhea, dietary adjustments are crucial. A diet rich in soluble fiber can help regulate bowel movements, while probiotic foods like yogurt can support gut health. On the other hand, avoiding high fiber foods and caffeine may be necessary for those experiencing diarrhea.

Weight management is another aspect of cancer nutrition that cannot be overlooked. Some patients may experience weight loss, while others may gain weight due to treatment related factors. Monitoring calorie intake and engaging in light physical activity, as tolerated, can help maintain a healthy weight.

Mouth sores and difficulty swallowing are painful side effects that can make eating difficult. Soft, soothing foods are often the best choice in this situation. Foods like yogurt, applesauce, mashed potatoes, and smoothies can be easier to swallow and less irritating to sore mouths.

Avoiding acidic, spicy, or rough textured foods can prevent further irritation. Drinking through a straw can help direct fluids away from painful areas in the mouth. Additionally, cold foods like ice cream or popsicles can numb the mouth and provide temporary relief from pain.

Bone health can also be affected by cancer treatments, particularly those that involve steroids or hormonal therapies. Ensuring adequate intake of calcium and vitamin D is crucial for maintaining bone strength. Dairy products, fortified plant based milks, leafy greens, and fish with bones (like sardines) are excellent sources of calcium. Vitamin D may be gained by sunshine, fatty fish, and fortified meals. In some cases, supplements may be necessary to ensure you're getting enough of these important nutrients.

The psychological impact of cancer treatment on eating habits is also significant. Food is not just nourishment; it's also associated with pleasure, social interactions, and emotional wellbeing. Creating a positive eating environment, involving family and friends in meal preparation, and focusing on the enjoyment of food can all contribute to a better eating experience.

It's important to remember that everyone's experience with cancer treatment is unique, and what works for one person may not work for another. Listening to your body and paying attention to how different foods make you feel can help you identify the best dietary choices for your specific needs. Keeping a food journal can be a helpful tool for tracking your intake and noting any patterns or changes in symptoms.

Fatigue: Strategies for Increased Energy Levels

"Energy and persistence conquer all things." – Benjamin Franklin

Fatigue is a common and often expected side effect of cancer and its treatment. It is a persistent, subjective sense of tiredness related to cancer or cancer treatment that interferes with usual functioning. Unlike the normal fluctuations of energy experienced by healthy individuals, cancer related fatigue is more severe, more distressing, and less likely to be relieved by rest. This type of fatigue can significantly impact a patient's quality of life, affecting physical, emotional, and cognitive functions.

For those undergoing cancer treatment, the management of fatigue is paramount. It involves a multifaceted approach that includes medical interventions, lifestyle modifications, and nutritional strategies. The latter, in particular, offers a no pharmacological avenue that can empower patients to take an active role in managing their symptoms.

Nutrition plays a critical role in combating fatigue. The body requires a variety of nutrients to produce energy and maintain muscle strength and endurance. During cancer treatment, the body's demand for energy and protein increases, making it essential to consume a diet that supports energy production and preserves muscle mass.

Protein is a key nutrient for energy and muscle maintenance. It is vital for the repair of body tissues and the immune system. Cancer patients should aim to include a source of protein with every meal and snack. Good sources of protein include lean meats, poultry, fish, eggs, dairy products, nuts, seeds, beans, and legumes.

Carbohydrates are the body's main source of energy. They should come primarily from complex carbohydrates, which provide a steady release of energy, rather than simple sugars that can lead to rapid spikes and drops in blood sugar levels.

Whole grains, fruits, vegetables, and legumes are excellent sources of complex carbohydrates that also provide fiber, vitamins, and minerals.

Healthy fats are also essential. They provide a concentrated source of energy and help with the absorption of fat soluble vitamins. Sources of healthy fats include avocados, nuts, seeds, olive oil, and fatty fish such as salmon, which is also high in omega3 fatty acids known for their anti-inflammatory properties.

Hydration is crucial as well, as even mild dehydration can exacerbate feelings of fatigue. Water, herbal teas, and broth based soups are good choices to maintain hydration levels.

Micronutrients, particularly B vitamins, vitamin D, iron, magnesium, and potassium, play significant roles in energy metabolism and muscle function. A diet rich in fruits, vegetables, whole grains, and lean proteins can help ensure adequate intake of these important nutrients.

Incorporating antioxidant rich foods into your diet can help combat inflammation and oxidative stress, both of which can contribute to fatigue. Berries, dark leafy greens, nuts, and seeds are rich in antioxidants. These foods can help protect your cells from damage and support your overall health during treatment.

Probiotic rich foods, such as yogurt, kefir, sauerkraut, and other fermented vegetables, can support gut health and improve digestion. A healthy gut microbiome is essential for nutrient absorption and overall energy levels. Including these foods in your diet can help maintain a balanced gut flora and support your immune system.

Creating a meal plan can help ensure you're consuming a balanced diet that supports your energy needs. Planning meals and snacks in advance can save time and reduce stress, making it easier to stick to a nutritious eating plan. Consider batch cooking and preparing meals in advance, so you have healthy options readily available even on days when you feel too tired to cook.

Counseling and support can be beneficial for managing the emotional and psychological aspects of fatigue. Speaking with a dietitian or nutritionist can provide personalized dietary advice and help develop meal plans that accommodate treatment schedules and side effects.

Complementary therapies such as yoga, massage, and acupuncture may also help reduce fatigue and improve energy levels. These therapies can complement conventional treatments by helping to reduce stress, improve sleep, and enhance overall wellbeing.

Maintaining a positive outlook and staying engaged in activities you enjoy can also help reduce fatigue. Pursuing hobbies, spending time with loved ones, and participating in social activities can provide a sense of normalcy and improve your emotional wellbeing. It's important to find joy in everyday activities and stay connected with your support network.

Remember that managing fatigue is an ongoing process, and it's important to be patient with yourself. Some days will be better than others, and that's okay. Consistently implementing these strategies and making adjustments as needed, you can improve your energy levels and enhance your quality of life during cancer treatment.

Nausea and Vomiting: Foods to Soothe and Support

"Food is the most primitive form of comfort." – Sheilah Graham Westbrook

Nausea and vomiting are among the most common and distressing side effects faced by cancer patients undergoing treatment. These symptoms can significantly impact a patient's ability to maintain adequate nutrition and hydration, which are crucial for healing and recovery.

The challenge, therefore, lies in identifying foods that not only soothe the stomach but also provide the necessary support to the body's nutritional needs.

The relationship between food and the management of nausea and vomiting is complex. Certain foods can help stabilize the stomach lining, reduce inflammation, and provide easy to digest nutrients that are less likely to exacerbate symptoms. The key is to focus on foods that are gentle on the stomach, appealing to the senses, and rich in nutritional value.

- **Bland Foods**: Starting with bland, starchy foods can be beneficial. Foods like toast, crackers, and pretzels are often recommended as they are easy to digest and unlikely to irritate the stomach1. These foods can also absorb stomach acids and are generally well tolerated even when nausea is at its peak.

- **Ginger:** Ginger is renowned for its anti-nausea properties. It can be consumed in various forms, such as ginger tea, ginger chews, or even raw ginger slices. The active components in ginger may help soothe the stomach and reduce the feeling of nausea.

- **Cold Foods**: Eating cold or room temperature foods can also be helpful as they tend to have less aroma, which can be beneficial if strong smells exacerbate nausea4. Foods like gelatin, popsicles, and cold fruit can be refreshing and less likely to trigger symptoms.

- **Hydration:** Staying hydrated is essential, especially if vomiting occurs. Small, frequent sips of clear liquids can prevent dehydration. Beverages like flat carbonated drinks, diluted fruit juices, and herbal teas can be soothing.

- **High Calorie Foods**: For patients struggling with weight maintenance, high calorie foods that are easy to eat can provide much needed energy. Options include pudding, ice cream, sherbets, yogurt, and milkshakes4. These can be consumed in small amounts throughout the day to help maintain calorie intake.

- **Protein:** Protein rich foods are important for healing and recovery. Boiled or baked meats, fish, and poultry; well cooked eggs; and low fat dairy products can be good sources of protein that are less likely to cause nausea.

- **Fruits and Vegetables**: Soft, bland fruits and vegetables like canned peaches or boiled potatoes can be included in the diet. They provide vitamins and minerals without causing undue stress on the digestive system.

- **Avoiding Irritants**: It is generally advised to avoid fatty, fried, spicy, or very sweet foods as they can be harder to digest and more likely to cause nausea.

- **Small Meals**: Eating small amounts often and slowly can help manage nausea. It's also beneficial to eat more of the foods that appeal to you and to eat in a place that is comfortable, avoiding stuffy places that are too warm or have cooking odors.

- **Rest:** Resting after eating and avoiding tightfitting clothes can also help reduce nausea. For morning nausea, eating crackers or toast before getting up can be effective

- **Medicinal Support**: While dietary strategies are important, it's also crucial to work with healthcare providers to manage nausea and vomiting through medication when necessary.

Recommended foods

- Creamed wheat, oatmeal, and cold cereal

- Soups

- Cold sandwiches.

- Cottage Cheese

- Hardboiled eggs.

- Plain spaghetti, rice, noodles, and mashed potatoes

- Toast and dry. Saltine crackers, natural potato chips, or pretzels

- Canned fruit, applesauce, and Jello

- Custard and Pudding

- Sherbet, popsicles, and frozen fruit bars

- Sodas, juices, and herbal teas

- Low fat protein sources, such as skinned chicken or tofu that is baked or broiled rather than fried.

- Peaches or other soft, mildly flavored fruits and vegetables

- Clear beverages such as apple and cranberry juice, low sodium broth, and fizzy drinks without caffeine

- Ginger and peppermint tea can be served lukewarm or cold.

Diarrhea and Constipation: Dietary Modifications for Relief

The digestive process and nutritional absorption rely heavily on the intestinal system, which is a symphony of muscle contractions and repetitive motions. However, cancer therapy can interrupt this delicate dance, resulting in unwanted visitors at either end of the digestive spectrum: diarrhea and constipation.

Constipation

Constipation can be caused by chemotherapy, certain drugs, or a lack of exercise. Including additional fiber in your diet may help. Here are some simple methods to increase fiber to your diet and relieve constipation.

- Consider include high fiber items in your diet, such as kidney beans, chickpeas, lentils, fresh fruit and vegetables, and dried fruit. Try to include fiber in all of your meals.
- Start your day with bran cereals or shredded wheat, or meals containing whole grains like bulgur or wheat berries. Aim for cereal that has at least 5 grams of fiber per serving.

- Combine unprocessed wheat bran with hot porridge and yogurt.

- If you aren't used to consuming a lot of fiber, gradually increase your consumption, since you may have more flatulence (gas) until your body adjusts to extra fiber in the diet.

- You may also minimize flatulence while eating beans by first soaking them in water and then discarding the water.

- Drink lots of drinks, eight to ten glasses every day. A high fiber diet requires lots of water to function properly.

- Reduce your caffeine intake, as it might cause constipation by causing you to lose fluids.

- When you wake up in the morning, drink a hot, caffeine free beverage like lemon water.

- Include exercise in your everyday regimen. Check with your doctor first.

Recommended foods

- Whole grain breads, pastas, and bran cereals
- Cooked beans, peas, and lentils
- Raw fruits and vegetables.
- Dried Fruit

- Prune juice and heated lemon water

Diarrhea

Diarrhea can have several causes. Chemotherapy, radiation therapy to the lower abdomen, malabsorption, or antibiotic usage are all potential causes. It may also occur as a result of milk intolerance or difficulties absorbing lipids. If you lose weight from diarrhea, it might be due to dehydration, which implies your body isn't getting enough water. Speak with your doctor to establish the reason of the weight loss and receive the appropriate therapy.

If you have diarrhea:

- Drink plenty of room temperature beverages to avoid dehydration. These might include water, teas, Gatorade, ginger ale, peach or apricot nectar, or fruit juices. Limit your intake of caffeine containing drinks.
- Allow carbonated drinks to lose their fizz or mix them before drinking.
- Eat more potassium rich foods like orange juice, tomato juice, bananas, and potatoes.
- Try the BRAT diet, which includes bananas, rice, applesauce, tea, and toast.

- Make frequent, modest meals.

- Avoid fried and greasy meals. Consume spicy or strongly seasoned foods only when tolerated.

- Reduce your consumption of fiber rich foods including whole grains, bran cereals, and veggies.

- Try breads made with oat flour or refined flour that include no seeds or nuts.

- Avoid raw vegetables, as well as unpeeled fruit's skins, seeds, and stringy fibers.

- Once the diarrhea has subsided, you can resume eating more fiber rich meals, fruits, and vegetables.

- If you are lactose sensitive, consume dairy products sparingly. Instead of ordinary milk, consider Lactaid, yogurt, or soy milk.

- Probiotics, glutamine, and/or digestive enzymes may help relieve symptoms. Please consult with a nutritionist about the usage of these supplements to see whether they are appropriate and which brands you should consider.

- Milk, ice cream, and puddings should be avoided for the time being since they might cause stomach trouble. Yogurt, sherbet, cheese, and custard may be tolerated because they contain less lactose.

Recommended foods

- Cream of wheat, oatmeal, plain rice, and maize cereals.

- Canned fruit, nectar, and applesauce

- White rice, spaghetti, and skinless potatoes

- Sandwiches with white bread

- Soups without cream.

- Cheese and crackers, graham crackers with peanut butter

- Eggs

- Jell-O with Popsicles

- Soda, herbal tea

- Nutritional beverages such as Ensure, Resource, Sustacal, Pediasure, and Boost.

Mouth Soreness: Choosing Comforting and Nutritious Options

"Food should be a comfort, not a challenge." –

Anonymous

"The human body," observed Epicurus, "is not clothed in silk and satin. It is clothed in skin." In the context of cancer treatment, this quote takes on a new dimension.

The delicate lining of your mouth, the gateway to your digestive system, can become a battleground during treatment. Mouth sores, also known as mucositis, are a prevalent and often debilitating side effect, affecting up to 40% of patients undergoing chemotherapy or radiation therapy. These painful lesions can significantly impact your ability to eat, speak, and swallow, jeopardizing your nutritional intake and overall wellbeing.

However, with careful selection and preparation of food, it is possible to not only soothe the soreness but also ensure that the body receives the nutrients it needs to heal and thrive during treatment.

While treatment is the primary culprit, other factors can exacerbate mouth sores:

- **Poor Oral Hygiene**: Inadequate oral hygiene practices like infrequent brushing and flossing can create a breeding ground for bacteria, increasing the risk of infection and worsening mouth sores.
- **Dehydration:** Dehydration can dry out the mouth, making it more susceptible to irritation and the development of sores.

- **Certain Medications**: Some medications, including diuretics and some pain medications, can contribute to dry mouth and increase the risk of mouth sores.

While mouth sores may be unavoidable, proactive measures can significantly reduce their severity and duration:

- **Maintain Excellent Oral Hygiene**: Brush your teeth with a soft bristled toothbrush and a gentle fluoride toothpaste at least twice a day, and floss gently once a day. Consider using a mouthwash specifically formulated for sensitive mouths, avoiding alcohol based rinses that can be drying.

- **Hydration is Key**: Stay well hydrated throughout the day by sipping on cool liquids like water, sugar free clear broths, or electrolyte replenishing beverages.

- **Schedule Regular Dental Checkups**: Inform your dentist about your cancer treatment and schedule regular checkups to monitor your oral health and address any potential issues early on.

The goal of managing mouth soreness is twofold: to minimize discomfort and to maximize nutritional intake. Foods that are soft, smooth, and easy to swallow can be particularly comforting.

These include items such as oatmeal, mashed potatoes, scrambled eggs, and well cooked pasta. Such foods require less chewing, reducing the risk of irritating sensitive mouth tissues.

Soft, easy to swallow foods are the cornerstone of a diet for those experiencing mouth soreness. These foods minimize irritation and are easier to consume. Examples include mashed potatoes, yogurt, applesauce, and scrambled eggs. Smoothies are an excellent option as they can be packed with nutrients and are easy to swallow. You can blend fruits, vegetables, protein powder, and healthy fats like avocado or nut butter to create a nutritious and soothing meal.

Milk and milk alternatives, such as almond milk or oat milk, can be soothing to a sore mouth. They are also a good source of protein and calcium, which are essential for maintaining your strength and bone health during treatment. You can use these in smoothies, or enjoy them on their own. Puddings and custards made with milk or milk alternatives can also be comforting and easy to eat.

Foods that are rich in protein are essential for healing and maintaining muscle mass. Soft proteins like cottage cheese, tofu, and scrambled eggs are gentle on the mouth.

You can also try soft cooked fish or chicken that has been finely chopped or blended into a smooth consistency. Incorporating protein into every meal and snack can help ensure you meet your nutritional needs.

Avoiding acidic, spicy, and rough textured foods is important when managing mouth soreness. These types of foods can irritate the mouth and exacerbate pain. Citrus fruits, tomatoes, and vinegar based dressings are examples of acidic foods that should be limited. Spicy foods, such as those containing hot peppers, can cause additional discomfort. Instead, opt for mild flavored foods that are gentle on the mouth.

Using a straw to drink liquids can help direct fluids away from sore areas in your mouth, reducing irritation. This can be particularly helpful when consuming beverages that might otherwise cause discomfort. Be sure to choose wide, flexible straws that are gentle on the mouth and lips.

Eating small, frequent meals can be more manageable than trying to consume large meals. This approach helps ensure you're getting enough calories and nutrients throughout the day without overwhelming your sore mouth. Keeping nutritious snacks within reach can make it easier to eat when you feel hungry.

Using soothing and moisturizing foods can help alleviate mouth soreness. Foods like gelatin, ice cream, and sorbet can provide temporary relief from pain. Ensure that these foods are not too cold, as extreme temperatures can sometimes increase sensitivity. Honey is another natural remedy that can help soothe a sore mouth. You can mix honey into warm tea or yogurt for a comforting treat.

Maintaining adequate nutrition is essential during cancer treatment, as it supports your body's ability to heal and fight infection. If you find it difficult to consume enough food due to mouth soreness, nutritional supplements may be helpful. These supplements can provide concentrated calories, protein, and other essential nutrients in a liquid or powdered form that is easier to swallow. Discuss with your healthcare provider to find the right supplement for your needs.

Soreness and discomfort in the mouth and throat are not unusual. If your swallowing issues are modest, the following recommendations may be useful. If you have serious issues, you may need to consult a nutritionist or swallowing therapist, as well as investigate other eating options.

- Consume frequent little meals and snacks to ensure that you are getting adequate calories. Select cold, smooth, and bland meals. Soft solids and liquids perform well.

- Cut or crush meals into bite sized bits to reduce the amount of chewing necessary.

- Soft meals or foods that can be cooked until tender include mashed potatoes, sweet potatoes, winter squashes (butternut and acorn), carrots, applesauce, ground beef or turkey, and tofu.

- Consume liquid supplements like Prosure, Ensure Plus, and Boost Plus, as well as smoothies mixed using a blender.

- Consider using a blender to purée the items your family eats. When adding liquid to process the items, use high calorie liquids like gravy, milk, soy milk, or broth instead of water.

- Drink plenty of healthful drinks with meals.

- Be adventurous. Try various sauces, gravies, or oils on dishes to make swallowing easier.

- If you are sensitive to citrus drinks, choose apple, cranberry, or grape juices, as well as fruit nectars.

- Keep some baby food on hand for fast and pleasant meals.

- Try sipping liquids with a straw or as directed by your swallowing therapist.
- Avoid spicy, salty, and acidic meals and drinks.

Recommended foods

- Nectar with apple juice
- Canned fruit and applesauce.
- Cream of Wheat
- Potato soup, chicken noodle soup, rice soup (juk)
- Custard, puddings, yogurt, and Jello
- Popsicle, ice cream, and sherbet
- Milkshakes & Carnation Instant Breakfast
- Nutritional beverages such as Ensure, Resource, Sustacal, Pediasure, and Boost.

Taste Changes: Adapting Your Diet for Enjoyment

"One cannot think well, love well, or sleep well if one has not dined well," Virginia Woolf said. But what happens when the very act of dining loses its appeal? Up to 70% of cancer patients undergoing treatment report experiencing taste changes, a condition known as dysgeusia.

This common side effect can significantly impact your appetite and enjoyment of food, making it challenging to maintain adequate nutrition.

Taste changes during cancer treatment can manifest in various ways. You might find that foods you once enjoyed now taste bland, metallic, or overly sweet or salty. Some patients experience a complete loss of taste (ageusia) or altered taste sensations. These changes can be caused by chemotherapy, radiation, medications, or the cancer itself. They can lead to decreased appetite, reduced food intake, and subsequent nutritional deficiencies. Addressing these taste changes is essential for maintaining your nutritional health.

One of the first steps in managing taste changes is to experiment with different flavors and textures. Foods that you previously enjoyed might no longer be appealing, so it's important to be open to trying new things. For example, if meat tastes metallic, try marinating it in acidic ingredients like lemon juice or vinegar to mask the metallic taste. Alternatively, you might find that plant based protein sources such as beans, lentils, or tofu are more palatable.

Flavor enhancers can also play a significant role in improving the taste of your food. Herbs and spices can add depth and complexity to your meals without overwhelming your taste buds. Fresh herbs like basil, cilantro, and mint can brighten flavors, while spices like cinnamon, turmeric, and cumin can add warmth and richness. Experiment with various combinations to determine what works best for you.

Texture is another important consideration when dealing with taste changes. You might find that certain textures are more appealing than others. For example, if you're experiencing a dry mouth, moist and juicy foods like stews, soups, and smoothies might be more enjoyable. On the other hand, if you have a heightened sensitivity to certain textures, you might prefer smoother, creamier foods like mashed potatoes, yogurt, and custards.

The temperature of your food can also affect how it tastes. Some patients find that cold or room temperature foods are more palatable than hot foods, which can have stronger odors and flavors. Cold dishes like salads, sandwiches, and chilled soups can be refreshing and easier to tolerate. Additionally, sucking on ice chips or frozen fruit popsicles before meals can help numb your taste buds and make eating more comfortable.

Taste fatigue can occur when you eat the same foods repeatedly, leading to a lack of enjoyment and decreased appetite. To combat this, try to incorporate a variety of foods into your diet. Rotating different cuisines and ingredients can keep your meals interesting and enjoyable. For example, you might have Italian one night, Mexican the next, and then Asian inspired dishes another night. This variety can help prevent boredom and make eating more pleasurable.

If you're experiencing a bitter or metallic taste, especially after chemotherapy, consider using plastic utensils instead of metal ones. This simple switch can sometimes reduce the metallic taste in your mouth. Additionally, drinking through a straw can help direct liquids past your taste buds, minimizing unpleasant flavors.

Maintaining good oral hygiene is crucial when dealing with taste changes. A clean mouth can improve your sense of taste and make eating more enjoyable. Brush your teeth and tongue gently with a soft bristled toothbrush and a mild toothpaste. Rinsing your mouth with a baking soda and water solution (1/4 teaspoon of baking soda in 1 cup of water) several times a day can help neutralize unpleasant tastes and keep your mouth fresh.

Mouth rinses designed specifically for cancer patients can also be effective in managing taste changes. These rinses can help soothe your mouth, reduce inflammation, and improve your ability to taste. Consult with your healthcare provider to find a suitable mouth rinse for your needs. They can also offer practical tips and strategies for managing taste changes and ensuring you're meeting your nutritional requirements.

Chapter 6: Building a Strong Immune System with Food

"The doctor of the future will interest his patients in the care of the human structure, food, and the cause and prevention of disease rather than giving them drugs," prophesied Thomas Edison.

Cancer treatment, while lifesaving, can take a toll on your immune system, your body's natural defense network. A weakened immune system leaves you more susceptible to infections and complications, potentially hindering treatment progress and impacting your overall wellbeing.

The immune system is an intricate network of cells, tissues, and organs that band together to defend the body against invaders. Those invaders can include bacteria, viruses, parasites, and even a fungus, all with the potential to make us sick. But what happens when the very treatments designed to target cancer also inadvertently weaken the immune system? This is where the power of food steps in, offering a beacon of hope and a tangible way to enhance one's defense mechanisms.

The immune system is a complex network of cells, tissues, and organs that cooperate to protect the body against dangerous intruders. Key components of this system include white blood cells, antibodies, and the lymphatic system. Nutrition plays a significant role in supporting these components, and a well-balanced diet can enhance your immune response. The right foods can be a source of strength, fortifying the body's natural defenses and providing the energy needed to endure the rigors of treatment. Conversely, the wrong dietary choices can deplete the immune system, leaving the body vulnerable to infections and complications.

Understanding the Immune System's Role in Cancer

Every second of the day, a fight between good and evil rages within your body. The immune system is beneficial since it is made up of armies of cells that protect the body against disease and infection. Pathogens, viruses, bacteria, and altered cells designed to do harm are the source of evil.

When the body battles cancer, the good guys do not always win. Healthy cells require a complex mix of internal and external signals between enzymes and proteins to function properly and control growth and division.

When such signals fail, the cells may run wild and expand out of control, resulting in a tumor.

The immune system defends the body from illnesses and infections caused by bacteria, viruses, fungus, or parasites. It is a set of reactions and responses that the body has to damaged cells or an infection. It is sometimes referred to as the immunological response.

People with cancer rely heavily on their immune systems because:

- Cancer may damage the immune system.
- Cancer therapies may damage the immune system.
- The immune system may help fight cancer.

Cancer and therapies might impair immunity

Cancer can compromise the immune system by infiltrating the bone marrow. Open a glossary item. The bone marrow produces blood cells, which aid in the fight against infection. This occurs most commonly in leukemia or lymphoma, although it can also occur in other malignancies. Cancer can prevent the bone marrow from producing as many blood cells.

Certain cancer therapies may temporarily impair the immune system. This is because they can induce a decrease in the quantity of white blood cells produced by the bone marrow. The following cancer therapies are more likely to damage the immune system:

- Chemotherapy
- Targeted cancer medications.
- Radiotherapy
- Massive doses of steroids.

The immune system can assist fight cancer

Some immune cells can identify cancer cells as aberrant and destroy them. However, this may not be enough to completely eliminate cancer. Some therapies attempt to employ the immune system to combat cancer.

The immune system consists of two fundamental parts:

- The protection we have since birth (inbuilt immunological defense)
- Acquired immunity is the protection we obtain after contracting certain illnesses.

Inbuilt immunological protection

This is also known as innate immunity. These processes are constantly alert and prepared to defend the body against infection. They can respond right away (or very rapidly). This inbuilt protection derives from:

The body's defense mechanisms include a skin barrier, mucus producing gut and lung linings, hairs that move mucus out of the lungs, stomach acid to kill bacteria, beneficial bacteria in the bowel to prevent overgrowth, urine flow to flush bacteria out of the bladder and urethra, and neutrophils to detect and kill bacteria.

Certain cancer therapies can also bypass these defense systems. Chemotherapy might temporarily lower the amount of neutrophils in your body, making it difficult to fight infections. Radiotherapy to the lungs can harm the hairs and mucus producing cells that assist to eliminate pathogens.

Neutrophils

Neutrophils are a kind of white blood cell that plays a crucial role in combating illness. They can do:

- Locate and adhere to infected regions of the body, including bacteria, viruses, and fungus.

- Gobble up the bacteria, viruses, or fungus and destroy them with chemicals.
- When you don't have enough neutrophils in your blood, your doctor may diagnose you as neutropenic.

Chemotherapy, targeted cancer medicines, and some radiation therapies can reduce the amount of neutrophils in the blood. As a result, following these therapies, you may develop new bacterial or fungal infections.

When undergoing cancer therapy, you should be aware of the following information:

- In those with low neutrophil counts, infections can become severe very fast.
- If you have a fever or feel unwell, get medical attention immediately.
- If your blood levels are low, antibiotics may be necessary to avoid serious infection.

It is more common to fall unwell from bugs that you carry with you than from catching someone else's. This implies that you should not have to avoid contact with your family, friends, or children following therapy.

Acquired immunity

This is immunological protection that the body develops after contracting certain illnesses. When the body encounters a new bacterium, fungus, or virus, it learns to identify it. So the next time the same bug invades the body, the immune system will have an easier job fighting it. This is why infectious illnesses like measles and chickenpox are often only contracted once.

Vaccination works by using this form of immunity. A vaccination comprises a little quantity of disease specific protein. This is not dangerous, but it helps the immune system detect the illness if it encounters it again. The immune reaction can then prevent you from contracting the illness.

Some vaccinations include tiny quantities of live germs or viruses. These are live, attenuated vaccinations. It implies that scientists modified the virus or bacterium such that it encourages the immune system to produce antibodies. A live vaccination will not transmit an infection.

Other vaccines make use of deceased bacteria or viruses, as well as protein fragments produced by bacteria and viruses.

B and T cells

Lymphocytes are a kind of white blood cell that participates in the acquired immune response. There are two major kinds of lymphocytes:

- B cells
- T cells

The bone marrow generates all blood cells, including B and T lymphocytes. They, like all other blood cells, must develop completely before they may contribute to the immune response.

B cells develop in the bone marrow. However, T lymphocytes develop in the thymus gland. Open a glossary item. Once mature, B and T cells move to the spleen. Open a glossary item, lymph nodes. Open a glossary item to combat infection.

Our lymphatic system and cancer page includes information about the thymus, spleen, and lymph nodes.

What do B cells do?

B cells respond to invading bacteria or viruses by producing proteins known as antibodies. Your body produces various antibodies for each type of germ (bug).

The antibody binds to the surface of the invading bacterium or virus. This labels the intruder so that the body recognizes it as hazardous and must be destroyed. Antibodies can also identify and eliminate damaged cells.

B cells contribute to the immune system's memory. The next time the same germ attempts to infiltrate, the B cells that produce the appropriate antibody are ready. They may produce their antibodies quite fast.

How do antibodies work?

Antibodies have two ends. One end adheres to proteins on the surface of white blood cells. The other end adheres to the germ or damaged cell, aiding in its eradication. The end of the antibody that binds to the white blood cell is always the same. Scientists refer to this as the "constant end."

The end of the antibody that detects germs and damaged cells differs depending on the cell it must recognize. So it is known as the changeable end. Each B cell produces antibodies with a different variable end than other B cells.

Cancer cells are not normal cells. So certain antibodies with different ends recognize and adhere to cancer cells.

What do T cells do?

There are two types of T cells called:

- Helper T cells
- Killer T cells

Helper T cells boost the production of antibodies by B cells and aid the development of killer cells.

Killer T cells eliminate the body's own cells that have been infected by viruses or bacteria. This inhibits the germ from replicating within the cell and infecting additional cells.

Does the immune system combat cancer?

Why do over two million Americans get cancer each year if their immune systems are so robust and sophisticated?

It might not be due to immune system problems. In reality, your immune system may be fighting cancer or pre cancer on a daily basis without your knowledge.

"The immune system is absolutely critical in fighting cancer," says Dr. Lynch.

Furthermore, the immune system is better suited to combating foreign cells that enter the body from outside, such as bacterial and viral infections.

Cancer cells are the body's own cells that have gone renegade, and the immune system may not recognize them as a threat.

Cancer cells frequently grow due to:

- Evade or hide from immune cells by employing signals that healthy cells can use.
- Shut down immune cells and occasionally employ them for proliferation.
- Overwhelm or exhaust the immune system with sheer numbers and fast expansion.

The burden of cell mutation and the immune system's ability to combat it strike a delicate balance. The point at which cancer begins to overpower the immune system is not usually clear.

"There are numerous reasons why that could happen," Dr. Lynch explains. "Some of it has to do with the tumor's DNA. Some of it is due to the cancer's aggressive nature."

According to research, cancer cells have enormous control over some innate and adaptive immune cells, which they exploit or recruit to grow and spread throughout the body. Because cancer cells are the body's own renegade cells, they know just which signals to transmit to mislead immune cells.

For example, regulatory T cells (Tregs) function as the immune system's off switch. They are intended to monitor an immune response and shut it off after the harmful cells have been eliminated.

However, Japanese researchers have found that cancer cells can deceive Tregs into suppressing the immune response, allowing the malignancy to spread.

Researchers have also discovered that cancer cells use long, hollow threads known as nanotubes to remove materials from the mitochondria of T cells, effectively sucking their vitality away.

Scientists face the issue of strengthening immune cells against cancer without inducing an autoimmune illness or causing a "cytokine storm" that permits the immune system to begin attacking healthy cells.

How might cancer immunotherapy help?

You may improve your immune system by eating a good diet, getting enough restful sleep, and exercising. However, such actions, together with others, may be insufficient to aid the body's battle against cancer.

With some malignancies, the immune system may need to be activated or boosted in order to better respond to cancer cells and detect them as harmful cells that must be removed.

Enter immunotherapy

Immunotherapy medications assist the immune system to discriminate between cancerous and normal cells. Immunotherapy medications are classified into several groups, some of which are given below.

- **Checkpoint inhibitors**: These medications are intended to interrupt the signals that cancer cells employ to elude the immune system.

- **Cytokines** are natural proteins that are created and supplied to control and direct the immune system's onslaught on cancer cells.

- **Vaccines**: Unlike flu shots and other disease prevention inoculations, cancer vaccines utilize medications to lower the risk of cancer by fighting cancer causing viruses or stimulating the immune system in a specific portion of the body.

CAR T cells, or chimeric antigen receptor T cells, are immune cells that have been taken from the blood and reengineered to attack cancer cells before being reintroduced to the body.

Immunotherapy medications do not directly destroy cancer cells, like chemotherapy and radiation treatment do. Instead, they activate the body's potent immune system.

"Immunotherapy is not going in there and killing the cancer cells," explains Dr. Lynch. "It's simply pulling the disguise off the cancer cell that's trying to hide and allowing the immune system to recognize it and do the job it's designed to do."

Dietary Strategies to Enhance Immune Function

Immunotherapy is emerging as a promising avenue in oncology, gaining increasing importance and offering substantial advantages when compared to chemotherapy or radiotherapy.

However, in the context of immunotherapy, there is the potential for the immune system to either support or hinder the administered treatment.

The immune system is the body's defense against infection and disease. It is a complex system that involves many different types of cells and molecules working together to protect the body.

Nutrition plays a critical role in immune function because many of the cells and molecules involved in the immune response require specific nutrients to function properly. For example, immune cells such as T cells and B cells require amino acids, which are the building blocks of protein, to function properly. Vitamin A is essential for the development and function of immune cells, and vitamin C is involved in the production of antibodies, which help to fight infection.

Dietary patterns and immune function

In addition to particular nutrients, dietary patterns can influence immune function. For example, the Mediterranean diet, which includes fruits, vegetables, whole grains, and healthy fats, has been found to have anti-inflammatory properties and may boost immune function. Diets heavy in saturated fat and sugar, on the other hand, have been found to promote inflammation and decrease immunological function. These eating habits have been related to an increased risk of chronic illnesses including obesity, type 2 diabetes, and cardiovascular disease, all of which are connected with weakened immune systems.

Nutritional treatments and immunological function

Nutritional treatments, such as taking supplements or eating fortified meals, can potentially have an influence on immunological function. For example, research has shown that vitamin D administration can boost immune function and lower the risk of respiratory infections. Zinc supplementation has also been proven to increase immunological function, particularly in elderly persons. Probiotics, which are living microorganisms that improve health, have also been examined for their immune boosting properties. Certain probiotic strains have been found in studies to boost immune function and lower the risk of respiratory infections.

The effect of diet on illness outcomes

Nutrition can also influence illness outcomes, especially in people with impaired immune systems. Individuals with Human Immunodeficiency Virus (HIV)/Acquired Immunodeficiency Syndrome (AIDS) have a weaker immune system and are more susceptible to infection. Proper eating is essential for these people since it helps to maintain immune function and lowers the risk of illness.

Similarly, cancer patients frequently have decreased immune function as a result of chemotherapy or radiation therapy. Nutritional measures, such as the use of vitamins or fortified meals, can assist these patients maintain immunological function and lower their susceptibility to infections.

Nutritional immunology is a burgeoning topic of research that investigates the link between nutrition and the immune system. It has grown in importance in recent years as researchers have become more interested in how diet might help prevent and treat disease.

Nutrition is crucial for immune function because many of the cells and molecules involved in the immunological response require certain nutrients to operate effectively. Dietary patterns and nutritional treatments can both influence immune function and illness consequences. More study is needed to completely understand the complicated interaction between diet and immune function, but current studies indicate that appropriate nutrition is essential for sustaining immune function and lowering the risk of infections and chronic illnesses.

Foods Rich in Immune Boosting Nutrients

Consuming a range of vitamin and mineral rich foods on a regular basis, such as citrus fruits, spinach, red peppers, and ginger, may assist to strengthen your immune system.

Natural immune boosters are things that we come across in our daily lives. The first line of defense is always a healthy lifestyle, which includes quitting smoking, eating enough of fruits and vegetables, exercising, getting enough sleep, and reducing stress. Humans have a long history of employing natural immune boosters in their daily lives, and this trend is growing as the adverse effects of synthetic medications become more common.

Water

Drinking plenty of water is beneficial for a variety of reasons, one of which is to reduce your risk of sickness. Staying hydrated helps nutrients to reach all areas of the body and keeps all biological systems and organs working properly, potentially lowering the risk of sickness. An adequate amount of water keeps the mucous membranes moist, lowering the incidence of colds and flu.

Drinking water helps to oxygenate cells, which leads to well-functioning systems. Well oxygenated cells are more suited to combating germs and other infectious agents than cells with low oxygen levels.

Furthermore, when someone is unwell, the body loses a lot of water in the form of mucus, which is used to eliminate infection causing bacteria. Water plays an important function in eliminating toxins from the body by transporting them via the kidneys and urinary system.

Dehydration can cause toxins to build up in the circulation and other important organs, resulting in a compromised immune system. Drinking enough of water throughout the day can assist to prevent dehydration and improve detoxification. Staying hydrated is also important for detoxification pathways, lymphatic drainage, and eliminating foreign invaders and debris.

Dehydration can lead to muscle tension, headaches, low serotonin levels, and digestive issues. Drinking more water can improve health both directly and indirectly by increasing urine flow or dilution and decreasing levels of osmotically induced vasopressin (AVP).

Elevated levels of circulating AVP have been linked to metabolic abnormalities, autosomal dominant polycystic kidney disease, and chronic kidney disease. In contrast, greater urine flow caused by consuming more water can help avoid kidney stones and minimize the recurrence of urinary tract infections.

Plant Based Foods

- Citrus fruits

The most popular citrus fruits include grapefruit, oranges, clementine, tangerines, lemons, and limes. Vitamin C, an essential vitamin present in citrus fruits, strengthens the immune system by increasing both adaptive and innate immune cells activity. It improves the epithelial barrier's ability to protect against infections.

Vitamin C may also promote the growth of infection fighting white blood cells known as lymphocytes and phagocytes, particularly the differentiation and proliferation of B and T cells, two of the immune system's most critical components.

It can also help prevent and treat respiratory and systemic infections. Vitamin C is also known to act as an antioxidant, helping to fight free radicals that damage and weaken the immune system's capacity to function properly.

Because the human body cannot produce or keep vitamin C, it is vital to consume high quality vitamin C sources on a regular basis, especially if one is ill, as vitamin C levels may be further reduced. Apart from vitamin C, citrus fruits include carotenoids, folic acid, dietary fibers, potassium, selenium, and a range of phytochemicals, making them a potent natural cancer fighting agent.

Citrus fruits include flavonoids, which function as anti-inflammatory and antioxidant agents, boosting the immune system by lowering inflammation and promoting faster recovery from disease. Naringin, a flavonoid present in citrus fruits, has been proven to inhibit the production of pro inflammatory cytokines. In addition to naringin, lemons contain Limonene, which can benefit the immune system.

Furthermore, the antioxidants included in lemons can help protect the eyes from age related damage such macular degeneration, as well as prevent cancer and cardiovascular disease.

- Papaya

Papaya is high in retinol, thiamine, riboflavin, niacin, folic acid, iron, potassium, calcium, and fiber, but low in calories. It includes carotenoids like βcarotene and lycopene, enzymes like chymopapain and papain, and antioxidants like vitamin C, which have been found to reduce the severity of ailments including rheumatoid arthritis, osteoarthritis, and asthma. βcarotene, a precursor of vitamin A, acts as an antioxidant and boosts immunological function. Vitamin A has been demonstrated to boost the immune system and aid in the development, reproduction, and synthesis of blood cells.

Furthermore, retinoic acid, a Vitamin A derivative, has been shown to stimulate the proliferation of lymphocytes and T cells at the site of inflammation in the stomach. It is important for a proper innate immune response. Vitamin A deficiency has been associated to decreased killer cell and eosinophil activity, as well as reduced neutrophil and macrophage oxidative burst and phagocytic capability.

- Kiwi

There are three varieties of commercial kiwi fruits: kiwi (Actinidia deliciosa), golden kiwi (Actinidia chinensis), and hardy kiwi (Actinidia arguta).

Kiwis, like papayas, provide critical nutrients such as potassium, vitamin C, carotenoids, fiber, vitamin K, and antioxidants. Kiwis have high quantities of vitamin C and polyphenols, which have anti-inflammatory properties that help regulate the immune system and lower the risk of influenza. In vitro studies have also demonstrated that golden kiwi can influence the immune system via modulating cell and cytokine activity.

- Pomegranate

Pomegranate juice has been found to suppress the development of dangerous bacteria, including E. coli O157:H7, Listeria, Shigella, Clostridium, Yersinia, Salmonella, and Staphylococcus aureus. It has also been demonstrated to have antiviral properties, making it useful against viruses like flu.

Pomegranate juice promotes the growth of healthy gut bacteria such as Bifidobacterium and Lactobacillus, which can significantly boost the immune system. Pomegranate intake lowers platelet aggregation, a key risk factor for cardiovascular disease. It also promotes good digestion, bowel movement, weight reduction, and overall immunity.

- Aonla

Aonla is a fruit high in vitamin C, flavonoids, and antioxidants that has been shown to have immunomodulatory and anti-inflammatory effects. Aonla contains ellagic acid, which is a potent antioxidant. Aonla has also been linked to increased natural killer cell activity and anti-body dependent cell cytotoxicity.

Aonla is a prospective candidate for cancer prevention and therapy due to its possible chemo modulatory, neuromodulatory, free radical scavenging, chemo preventive effects, antioxidant, anti-mutagenic, anti-inflammatory, and immunomodulatory capabilities. Aonla has high levels of vitamin C, flavonoids, and antioxidants, and it has been proven to have immunomodulatory and anti-inflammatory properties. Aonla contains ellagic acid, which is a potent antioxidant.

- Almonds

Almonds are high in vitamin E, which, like vitamin C, is necessary for a healthy immune system. Vitamin E is a powerful antioxidant that promotes healthy immunological function.

In addition to vitamin E, almonds include monounsaturated and polyunsaturated fats, flavonoids such as kaempferol, catechin, epicatechin, and isorhamnetin, and plant sterols. These components play critical roles in almonds' potential to influence immunological and inflammatory processes. Almonds have an anti-inflammatory impact on cardiovascular illnesses, and vitamin E in the body serves as an antioxidant. Vitamin E also plays an important role in T cell development.

- Broccoli

Broccoli is a green vegetable with a fleshy stalk and a huge blooming head that is eaten all over the world in many forms such as cooked vegetables, salad, soup, and so on. Broccoli is regarded as one of the healthiest vegetables available due to its high levels of vitamins A, C, and E, fiber, and antioxidants.

Broccoli's favorable benefits on human health are due to its high content of minerals, vitamins, and isothiocyanates, the most important of which is sulforaphane (SFN). SFN has been shown to have anti-inflammatory and cancer preventing properties. To keep its potential, broccoli should be consumed as little prepared as possible or uncooked.

Steaming is also one of the most effective ways to prepare foods while retaining nutritional value. Broccoli's health advantages extend beyond its nutritional value since it includes a variety of phytochemicals such as polyphenols, glucosinolates, and their derivatives, which include isorhamnetin, quercetin glucosides, and kaempferol. These components add to the vegetable's antioxidant and anticancer capabilities, making it a popular meal choice among health conscious people.

Furthermore, multiple epidemiological studies have validated broccoli's nutritional and therapeutic benefits, including its capacity to control immunity, aid in detoxification, boost eye and bone health, and possess antibacterial and antioxidant capabilities.

- Ginger

Ginger (Zingiber officinale Roscoe) is a common condiment used in many cuisines across the world. The rhizomes of ginger produce oleoresin, which includes multiple bioactive components, including gingerol, the principal pungent element thought to have exceptional pharmacological and physiological benefits.

Ginger is well known for its ability to boost appetite, promote digestion, function as a cold remedy, and provide analgesic and anti-inflammatory properties. Red ginger, which has more powerful bioactive chemicals than conventional ginger, has shown promise as an immunomodulatory in the treatment of psoriasis. Studies have indicated that red ginger can affect T lymphocyte activation.

In addition to its immunomodulatory characteristics, ginger has been demonstrated to offer potential advantages for chronic pain relief and cholesterol reduction. Excessive creation of reactive oxygen species (ROS) or free radicals during metabolism overwhelms a biological system's antioxidant capacity, resulting in oxidative stress, which has been linked to heart disease, cancer, neurological diseases, and the aging process.

Ginger's bioactive components, including gingerols, have been shown to exhibit antioxidant properties in a range of modules. Increased consumption of antioxidantrich foods and beverages, such as ginger shots, may help battle inflammation and keep the immune system healthy.

- Garlic

Garlic has been utilized as a popular plant cure in traditional medicine since antiquity. Freshly crushed garlic contains a high variety of physiologically active sulfur containing chemicals, such as sulfoxides, proteins, and polyphenols, which have been shown to have antiviral activities and to boost immunological function.

Garlic has been proven to have immunostimulant effects, which might be beneficial in medicinal applications. It stimulates innate and specific cell immunity by activating natural killer cells, lymphocytes, macrophages, dendritic cells, and eosinophils. These immune cells are known to increase immune system function, potentially lowering the risk of specific illnesses. Garlic includes the sulfoxide alliin, which, when crushed or swallowed, is transformed into allicin.

Furthermore, garlic's bioactive component diallyl sulfide (DAS) can inhibit inflammatory variables such as reactive oxygen species (ROS), NFkB (nuclear factor kappa light chain enhancer of activated B cells), and cyclooxygenase2 production via the NFkB pathway. This route is critical for cytokine generation and cell survival, therefore inhibiting it may assist to lessen inflammation.

In vitro studies have shown that garlic has antithrombotic properties and reduces platelet aggregation in people. Its components have been found to have a variety of immunomodulatory effects on leukocyte cytokine production. Garlic eating enhances hematological and homeostatic markers. Garlic eating may stimulate the production and release of nitric oxide (NO), which is responsible for increased interferon alpha release in humans and is useful against viral and proliferative disorders.

- Onion

Onion (Allium cepa L.) is a popular element in Indian cuisine and a globally farmed and consumed vegetable. Its use stretches back to ancient Egypt, when it was prized for its antibacterial, anti-inflammatory, and therapeutic characteristics. Onions' health advantages are linked to their bioactive components, which include organosulfur compounds like diallyl sulfide and diallyl sulfoxide, proteins, peptides, and flavonoids, namely quercetin derivatives. These chemicals provide onions with antioxidant, antibacterial, antiviral, antifungal, anti-carcinogenic, anti-inflammatory, and antimutagenic activities.

Onion fructooligosaccharides (FOS) have high mitogenic and phagocytic activity, implying a potential role in therapeutic immunomodulation.

- Turmeric

Turmeric, a bright yellow and bitter spice prevalent in curries, has been used as an anti-inflammatory to treat osteoarthritis and rheumatoid arthritis. Its primary component, curcumin, has been shown to help prevent exercise induced muscle damage due to its high yellow pigment content. Animal studies have also revealed that curcumin can improve immunity and has antiviral capabilities.

Curcumin, the main ingredient in turmeric, has been shown to regulate a variety of biological functions, including signal transducers, transcription factors, mitogen activated protein kinase, cytokine production, and immune cell receptors. It has been demonstrated to influence the activity of immune cells such as B cells, dendritic cells, monocytes, macrophages, and neutrophils, hence impacting both innate and adaptive immunity in pathological situations.

Curcumin is also renowned for its antioxidant characteristics, which include serving as an oxygen free radical scavenger, protecting hemoglobin from oxidation, and inhibiting microbe and viral proliferation.

- Green and black tea

Green and black teas contain high levels of flavonoids, an antioxidant. Green tea includes EGCG, an antioxidant that boosts immune function. EGCG stimulates the production of immune regulatory cytokines, lowers the risk of many illnesses, reduces inflammation, and protects cells from damage. The fermentation procedure used to create black tea destroys a significant portion of the EGCG, but green teas retain the EGCG since they are steamed rather than fermented.

Green tea is also high in theanine, an amino acid that may aid in the production of germ fighting chemicals in T cells. Tea preparations have antioxidant characteristics and contain phenolic chemicals such thearubigins and theaflavins, which have been demonstrated to have potential therapeutic benefits on cancer, cardiovascular disease, and inflammation. These chemicals have been identified for their antioxidant properties and other health advantages.

Herbal teas, as opposed to traditional teas prepared from Camellia sinensis leaves, are made out of a variety of dried plant components such as fruits, flowers, seeds, nuts, barks, and grasses, including chamomile, cinnamon, ginseng, ginger root, cardamom, parsley, and cloves, among others. These chemicals have immune boosting effects that might be useful to human health, such as anti-inflammatory, antiviral, anticancer, antioxidant, and antibacterial activity.

- Mushrooms

Mushrooms are edible fungus that contain high levels of selenium as well as B vitamins like niacin and riboflavin, all of which help strengthen the human immune system. Selenium, in particular, acts as an antioxidant, helping to minimize oxidative stress and inflammation while also boosting immunological function.

Vitamin B6 promotes communication between cytokines and chemokines, as well as enhancing immunological response to elevated antibody production. A shortage of vitamin B6 reduces lymphocyte growth and proliferation, antibody generation, and T cell activity. Mushrooms include bioactive chemicals that modulate the immune system, including βdglucan, polysaccharide peptide/protein complexes, proteins, proteoglycans, and triterpenoids.

βdglucan from mushrooms has been demonstrated to increase the immunological response of NK cells, B cells, T cells, and macrophages. They are also thought to have anti-cholesterol, anti-allergy, anticancer, and antitumor effects. Mushrooms have a multitude of effects, including the ability to stimulate cytokine production, which are small, soluble proteins that serve as intracellular mediators.

ANIMAL SOURCED FOODS

Animal sourced foods (ASF) are high in calories and provide high quality, readily digestible protein. The proteins in these meals are thought to be of the highest quality and easily available to the body since they include the whole set of necessary amino acids required by the human body. Animal based diets are also rich in micronutrients. Mild to severe protein energy malnutrition (PEM) is common in developing nations.

Malnutrition is particularly problematic for children since it leads to stunted growth, decreased mental development, and illness. Furthermore, the synergistic relationships between PEM, infection, and immune function are well documented. Given this, the inclusion of animal based foods such as milk, meat, eggs, and fish all contribute to a well-balanced human diet, especially in terms of immune function.

- Milk

Milk contains a variety of critical elements, including vitamins, minerals, and specific proteins, all of which are needed for overall health. Its immunological qualities have long been recognized; prolactin, a hormone found in milk, can promote lymphocyte and thymocyte migration, so enhancing immune function. Milk also includes immunoglobulins (IgA and IgG), which might influence the humoral immune response.

Furthermore, peptides and protein hydrolysates derived from milk's caseins and major whey proteins have immunomodulatory properties, such as enhancing lymphocyte proliferation, modulating cytokines, and promoting antibody production. Milk proteins (casein and whey) and milk fat account for the majority of bovine milk's immunomodulatory characteristics. Incorporating whey protein and αlactalbumin into the diet increases lymphocyte function and spleen generated lymphocytes' reactivity to T cell mitogens. Similarly, LF and CGP produced from Kcasein have been shown to increase lymphocyte function. In vitro tests suggest that peptides formed from enzymatic cleavage of α and βcasein can boost human lymphocyte function.

Fukushima et al. (2007) discovered that including fermented milk into the elderly's diet increased blood cell phagocytic activity. In addition to changing lymphocyte activity, dietary milk proteins have been shown to affect antibody responses. Using αlactalbumin, αlactalbumin hydrolysate, and whole whey protein concentrate leads to increased antibody production against foreign antigens. Golden milk, a milk based drink (half a teaspoon of turmeric powder in 150 mL hot milk), is said to boost immunity when eaten once or twice a day. Turmeric's major constituent, curcumin (Curcuma longa L.), regulates cytokine production, namely interleukin1, interleukin6, and tumor necrosis factorα.

Milk contains βCarotene, an antioxidant and precursor of vitamin A, which helps improve immunological function. It can protect phagocytic cells from oxidative damage, boost the activity of effector T cells, and improve the capacity of macrophages, cytotoxic T cells, and natural killer cells to destroy malignant cells. Vitamin A, generated from βCarotene, can improve epithelial tissue function, lymphoid mass, and immunity, thereby lowering the risk of infection.

- Yogurt & curd

Yogurt is a milk based food that is fermented by lactic acid bacteria (LAB), such as Lactobacillus bulgaricus and Streptococcus thermophilus. While milk and yogurt have comparable mineral compositions, certain elements, such as calcium, are better absorbed from yogurt than milk. Furthermore, yogurt has less lactose and more lactic acid, peptides, galactose, free fatty acids, and free amino acids than milk.

Several studies have shown that the therapeutic effects of LAB and yogurt, including their potential to enhance the immune system, are mostly due to changes in the micro ecology of the gastrointestinal tract. Yogurt eating can increase the population of LAB in the intestines, helping to prevent the growth of bad bacteria, resulting in fewer illnesses and more anticarcinogenic benefits. The amount to which LAB may activate the immune system is also determined by their closeness to lymphoid tissues when colonizing the intestinal lumen.

Consumption of curd has been demonstrated to improve human health, particularly the immune system. Curd can boost natural immunity by activating both mucosal and systemic host defenses.

This is accomplished by activating macrophages, increasing immunoglobulin levels, and enhancing natural killer cell activity and cytokine synthesis within the body. Regular yogurt eating can reduce the risk of cardiovascular disease, chronic renal disease, and diabetes while also strengthening the host's immune system.

- Egg

Eggs from domestic poultry birds are a low cost and commonly available food in many parts of the world. These are high in vitamins and minerals; nonetheless, there has been much dispute over whether eggs are healthy, particularly in terms of cholesterol. Eggs include protein, which is essential for the maintenance and repair of muscles and other physiological components.

Furthermore, eggs include vitamins and minerals that are required for normal brain and neurological function. Eggs are high in vitamin A, vitamin B12, and selenium, all of which aid to improve the immune system. Eggs include choline, which can help break down homocysteine, an amino acid related to heart disease. Finally, eggs include the antioxidants lutein and zeaxanthin, which help prevent age related macular degeneration.

Eggs are a great source of antioxidants and high quality proteins that are similar to those found in breast milk. Eggs include antioxidants (phosvitin and ovotransferrin), which inhibit lipid oxidation by metal chelation and arrest free radicals. Other vitamins included in eggs aid to preserve good vision.

Ovomucin, ovotransferrin, ovalbumin, avidin, and lysozyme are the main bioactive components of egg white with antibacterial properties. These proteins exert antibacterial and immunomodulatory actions via inflammatory pathways. As a result, including eggs into a regular diet may be a good choice for maintaining a balanced and healthy diet, particularly in impoverished areas where high value proteinaceous foods such as lentils and milk are not readily available.

Part 4:
Putting it All Together: Creating Your Personalized Plan

Chapter 7: Plans for different dietary preferences

Nutrition is essential for cancer management and therapy because it supports your immune system and general wellbeing. Varied patients have varied food preferences, and it is critical to learn how to customize nutrition regimens to fit their interests while still meeting all nutritional demands. Whether you eat vegetarian, vegan, or any other type of diet, there are strategies to maximize your nutritional intake to support your health throughout cancer treatment.

Vegetarians must ensure that they get adequate protein, iron, and vitamin B12, all of which are commonly found in animal products. Protein is necessary for muscle repair and immunological function and may be found in a number of plant based foods. Beans, lentils, and chickpeas are high protein legumes that may be used to soups, stews, salads, and main courses. Nuts and seeds, such as almonds, walnuts, chia seeds, and flaxseed, are high in protein and good fats. Dairy products and eggs, when incorporated in a vegetarian diet, give more protein, calcium, and vitamin B12.

Iron is another important mineral for vegetarians since plant based iron (nonheme iron) is not as easily absorbed by the body as iron from animal sources (heme iron). To improve iron absorption, combine iron rich meals with vitamin C rich foods. For example, add bell peppers, tomatoes, or citrus fruits to meals including spinach, tofu, or fortified cereals. Furthermore, cooking using cast iron cookware can boost the iron content of your meals.

Vitamin B12 is largely found in animal sources, therefore vegetarians, particularly vegans, may need to consider fortified meals or supplements. Fortified cereals, nutritional yeast, and plant based milks frequently include vitamin B12. Vitamin B12 levels should be monitored on a regular basis, and you should check with your doctor to ensure you are getting enough.

Those who adopt a vegan diet face comparable but more comprehensive issues owing to the elimination of all animal products. Protein consumption may be met via a number of plant based sources. Soy products like tofu, tempeh, and edamame, as well as legumes, nuts, and seeds, are high in protein. Whole grains including quinoa, bulgur, and farro also help with protein consumption.

It might be difficult to get enough calcium without dairy, but there are many of plant based options. Leafy greens like kale, collard greens, and bok choy are excellent choices. Fortified plant based milks, such as almond, soy, and oat milk, include more calcium and vitamin D. Tofu prepared with calcium sulfate and fortified orange juice are other feasible options.

Fish are high in omega3 fatty acids, which are beneficial to heart health and reduce inflammation. Vegans may get their omegas from flaxseeds, chia seeds, hemp seeds, and walnuts. Algal oil supplements are another great source of DHA and EPA, the active omegas found in fish.

A balanced diet rich in fruits and vegetables is essential for delivering the vitamins, minerals, and antioxidants required to boost the immune system, regardless of dietary choice. Berries, citrus fruits, leafy greens, cruciferous vegetables, and vividly colored fruits and vegetables are especially high in antioxidants and phytonutrients, which assist to counteract oxidative stress and promote general health.

Patients on a gluten free diet, whether due to celiac disease or gluten sensitivity, must be aware of hidden sources of gluten in processed goods. The diet should be built around whole foods like fruits and vegetables, lean meats, nuts and seeds, and gluten free grains like rice, quinoa, and millet.

Gluten free flours, such as almond flour, coconut flour, and chickpea flour, can be used in baking and cooking instead of wheat flour. It is critical to ensure that processed gluten free goods are nutrition rich and do not rely heavily on refined carbohydrates and sugars.

Those following a lowcarb or ketogenic diet seek to minimize carbohydrate intake while increasing fat consumption in order to achieve ketosis, a condition in which the body burns fat for fuel. This diet might be difficult to stick to after cancer treatment since it requires nutrient dense meals. No starchy veggies, high quality proteins, and healthy fats are all needed. Avocados, almonds, seeds, olive oil, coconut oil, and fatty fish are all good sources of healthful fat. No starchy vegetables such as leafy greens, broccoli, cauliflower, and zucchini are high in vitamins and minerals but low in carbs.

Patients on a paleo diet, which stresses whole, unprocessed foods and avoids grains, legumes, and dairy, can benefit from a wide range of nutrient rich foods. Lean meats, fish, eggs, fruits, vegetables, nuts, and seeds should be the primary focus. It is critical to ensure appropriate calcium consumption, which might be difficult without dairy.

Calcium rich foods include leafy greens, fish with bones, and fortified plant milks.

For people who follow certain cultural or religious dietary practices, such as kosher or halal diets, it is critical to ensure that all meals fit dietary restrictions while still being healthy and beneficial to health throughout cancer treatment. Kosher diets demand that meals be cooked in accordance with Jewish dietary restrictions, which include avoiding pork and shellfish and not combining meat and dairy. Halal diets require that meals be lawful under Islamic law, which includes avoiding pork and ensuring that meat is killed in accordance with certain criteria. Both dietary choices may contain a diverse range of fruits, vegetables, grains, and proteins that promote general health.

Regardless your food preferences, staying hydrated is critical. Water is essential to all body activities, including the immune system. Herbal teas, clear broths, and watery fruits and vegetables can all help you stay hydrated.

Regular, short meals throughout the day can help regulate hunger and provide constant nutritional intake. This method can reduce sensations of fullness or bloating associated with bigger meals, making it simpler to maintain enough nutrition during therapy.

Cooking at home using fresh, complete foods provides greater control over the nutritional value of meals. Simple, easy to prepare meals that cater to dietary requirements can make meal planning easier. For example, a vegetarian stir fry with tofu and a variety of colorful veggies is a well-balanced meal high in protein, vitamins, and minerals. A vegan lentil soup with carrots, celery, and tomatoes is a satisfying and nutrient dense alternative.

Meal planning and bulk cooking might save time and energy on days when you're feeling tired. Preparing big quantities of soups, stews, and casseroles and freezing them in individual servings will help you have healthful meals ready to eat. The labeling and timing of these meals assures their diversity and freshness.

Consider nutrient dense snacks that fit your dietary choices. Vegetarians and vegans may enjoy hummus with veggie sticks, nut butter on apple slices, or date and nut energy balls. Gluten free diet followers may pick rice cakes with avocado or gluten free granola bars. Lowcarb or ketogenic dieters may like cheese and nut mix, celery sticks with almond butter, or hardboiled eggs.

Incorporating nutrient dense smoothies can help you acquire a range of vitamins and minerals. A smoothie made with leafy greens, various fruits, a scoop of protein powder, and a splash of plant based milk may be customized to meet any nutritional needs. Adding flaxseeds, chia seeds, or spirulina can increase the nutritious value even further.

It's also critical to listen to your body and change your diet as necessary. Taste alterations, nausea, and other treatment related side effects might influence whether meals are attractive and tolerated. Being adaptable and willing to test new meals might help you identify the alternatives that work best for you at various phases of therapy.

Working with a registered dietician who specializes in cancer nutrition might give more tailored advice and assistance. A dietitian can help you create a dietary plan that is personalized to your unique needs, preferences, and treatment objectives. They can also provide practical advice and tactics for including immune boosting foods in your diet.

Meals catering to specific treatment phases

Building a strong immune system with food is a critical component of managing cancer and its treatment. The nutritional needs of cancer patients can vary significantly depending on the phase of treatment they are in. Here, I provide sample meal plans tailored to specific treatment phases to help you maintain optimal nutrition and support your immune system. Understanding how to adjust your diet during different phases of treatment can make a substantial difference in your overall wellbeing and recovery process.

Phase 1: Pre Treatment Nutrition

Before starting treatment, it is essential to strengthen your body with nutrient dense foods. The goal is to build up your immune system, maintain a healthy weight, and ensure you have the energy and nutrients needed to handle the upcoming treatment.

Breakfast:

- Smoothie with spinach, banana, blueberries, flaxseeds, and almond milk. Add a scoop of protein powder for extra protein.
- Whole grain toast with avocado and a poached egg.

- Oatmeal topped with chia seeds, sliced almonds, and fresh berries.

Lunch:

- Quinoa salad with mixed greens, cherry tomatoes, cucumbers, chickpeas, and a lemon tahini dressing.
- Lentil soup with carrots, celery, and tomatoes. Serve with a side of whole grain bread.
- Grilled chicken breast with a side of roasted sweet potatoes and steamed broccoli.

Dinner:

- Baked salmon with a quinoa and kale salad, dressed with a lemon vinaigrette.
- Stir-fried tofu with mixed vegetables (bell peppers, snow peas, carrots) served over brown rice.
- Spaghetti with whole grain pasta, marinara sauce, and turkey meatballs. Include a side of steamed asparagus.

Snacks:

- Greek yogurt with honey and walnuts.
- Apple slices with almond butter.
- Carrot sticks with hummus.

Phase 2: During Treatment Nutrition

During treatment, side effects such as nausea, vomiting, mouth sores, and fatigue can make eating challenging. The focus should be on easily digestible, high calorie, and high protein foods that are gentle on the stomach and easy to prepare.

Breakfast:

- Smoothie with banana, mango, spinach, Greek yogurt, and a touch of honey.
- Soft scrambled eggs with a side of mashed avocado on toast.
- Rice pudding made with coconut milk, cinnamon, and raisins.

Lunch:

- Creamy butternut squash soup with a side of soft whole grain bread.
- Mashed potatoes with grilled chicken and steamed green beans.
- Soft tofu stir fry with rice noodles and mild vegetables (zucchini, mushrooms).

Dinner:

- Baked cod with mashed sweet potatoes and a side of steamed spinach.
- Soft vegetable lasagna with layers of zucchini, ricotta cheese, and marinara sauce.
- Turkey and vegetable casserole with a creamy sauce.

Snacks:

- Cottage cheese with soft, canned peaches.
- Smoothies with almond milk, berries, and protein powder.
- Applesauce or fruit purees.

Phase 3: Post Treatment Nutrition

After treatment, the focus shifts to recovery and rebuilding strength. The diet should include foods that promote healing, restore energy, and boost the immune system.

Breakfast:

- Smoothie bowl with blended spinach, banana, and almond milk, topped with granola and fresh berries.
- Overnight oats with chia seeds, almond milk, and sliced bananas.
- Scrambled tofu with spinach and whole grain toast.

Lunch:

- Salmon and avocado salad with mixed greens, cherry tomatoes, and a balsamic vinaigrette.
- Chickpea and quinoa salad with roasted vegetables and a lemon tahini dressing.
- Turkey and vegetable wrap with hummus in a whole grain tortilla.

Dinner:

- Grilled shrimp with brown rice and steamed broccoli.
- Stuffed bell peppers with ground turkey, quinoa, and black beans.
- Roasted chicken with mashed cauliflower and sautéed kale.

Snacks:

- Protein bars with minimal sugar.
- Nut butter on whole grain crackers.
- Fresh fruit slices with Greek yogurt dip.

Phase 4: Long Term Maintenance Nutrition

Once treatment is completed, it is important to maintain a balanced diet to support long term health and prevent recurrence. Focus on a varied diet rich in fruits, vegetables, lean proteins, and whole grains.

Breakfast:

- Smoothie with kale, pineapple, chia seeds, and coconut water.
- Whole grain pancakes with fresh berries and a drizzle of maple syrup.
- Poached eggs on whole grain toast with a side of sautéed spinach.

Lunch:

- Grilled chicken salad with mixed greens, avocado, cherry tomatoes, and a honey mustard dressing.
- Lentil and vegetable stew with a side of whole grain bread.
- Quinoa bowl with black beans, corn, avocado, and a cilantro lime dressing.

Dinner:

- Baked salmon with a side of quinoa and roasted Brussels sprouts.
- Chicken and vegetable stirfry with brown rice.
- Vegetarian chili with kidney beans, black beans, and a variety of vegetables, served with cornbread.

Snacks:

- Trail mix with nuts, seeds, and dried fruit.
- Sliced cucumber and bell peppers with hummus.
- Greek yogurt with a sprinkle of granola and honey.

Special Considerations for Nutrient Dense Foods

Throughout all phases of treatment, it is crucial to incorporate nutrient dense foods that support the immune system and overall health. These foods include:

- **Leafy Greens**: Spinach, kale, and Swiss chard are rich in vitamins A, C, and K, as well as folate and iron.
- **Berries:** Blueberries, strawberries, and raspberries are high in antioxidants, which help combat oxidative stress and support the immune system.

- **Nuts and Seeds:** Almonds, walnuts, chia seeds, and flaxseeds provide healthy fats, protein, and fiber.

- **Lean Proteins:** Chicken, turkey, fish, tofu, and legumes are essential for muscle repair and immune function.

- **Whole Grains:** Brown rice, quinoa, oats, and whole wheat products offer fiber, B vitamins, and essential minerals.

- **Healthy Fats:** Avocados, olive oil, and fatty fish like salmon and mackerel support brain health and reduce inflammation.

Practical Tips for Meal Preparation

1. Batch Cooking: Prepare large quantities of soups, stews, and casseroles and freeze them in individual portions. This ensures you always have a nutritious meal on hand, even on days when cooking feels overwhelming.

2. Simple Recipes: Focus on recipes with minimal ingredients and straightforward preparation methods. Slow cookers and pressure cookers can be invaluable for making hearty meals with little effort.

3. Use High Quality Ingredients: Whenever possible, choose organic fruits and vegetables, lean cuts of meat, and whole grains. Quality ingredients can enhance the nutritional value and flavor of your meals.

4. Stay Hydrated: Alongside your meals, ensure you are drinking plenty of fluids. Water, herbal teas, and broths are excellent choices to maintain hydration and support your body's functions.

5. Listen to Your Body: Pay attention to how your body responds to different foods and adjust your diet accordingly. Some days you may crave hearty, comforting foods, while other days lighter, easy to digest options may be more appealing.

Incorporating Supplements

In some cases, dietary supplements may be necessary to meet your nutritional needs, especially if you are struggling with appetite loss or difficulty eating certain foods. Common supplements for cancer patients include:

- **Protein Powders:** To boost protein intake, consider adding protein powders to smoothies, oatmeal, or soups.

- **Multivitamins:** A high quality multivitamin can help fill any nutritional gaps in your diet.

- **Vitamin D**: If you have limited sun exposure or difficulty getting enough vitamin D from food, a supplement may be recommended.

- **Probiotics:** To support gut health, consider incorporating probiotic supplements or probiotic rich foods like yogurt and kefir.

Always consult with your healthcare provider before starting any new supplements to ensure they are appropriate for your specific needs and treatment plan.

Emotional and Social Aspects of Eating

Maintaining a positive attitude towards food and eating can significantly impact your overall wellbeing. Eating should be a pleasurable experience, not a chore. Here are some tips to make mealtimes more enjoyable:

1. Eat with Others: Sharing meals with family and friends can provide emotional support and make eating more enjoyable.

2. Create a Pleasant Eating Environment: Set the table, play some soft music, and take the time to savor your food.

3. Be Flexible: Some days you may not feel like eating much, and that's okay. Focus on nutrient dense snacks and small meals that you find appealing.

4. Celebrate Small Wins: Whether it's trying a new recipe, finishing a meal, or maintaining your weight, celebrate these achievements. Every step forward is a victory.

Building a strong immune system with food involves more than just eating the right nutrients; it's about creating a sustainable, enjoyable, and nourishing approach to eating that supports your body through every phase of cancer treatment.

Tips for Meal Prepping and Planning for Convenience

Meal prepping and planning are powerful strategies to help cancer patients maintain a strong immune system and manage their nutritional needs with ease and convenience. The process of planning and preparing meals in advance can reduce the stress and effort associated with daily cooking, ensuring that you have access to nutritious meals even on days when you feel tired or unwell. Here are some comprehensive tips for meal prepping and planning that will support your journey towards optimal health.

Understand Your Nutritional Needs

Before you begin meal prepping, it's essential to understand your specific nutritional needs. Cancer patients often require a diet that is high in protein, vitamins, and minerals to support immune function, muscle repair, and overall health. Consult with your healthcare provider or a registered dietitian to tailor your meal plan according to your treatment phase, symptoms, and personal preferences.

Plan Your Meals around Nutrient Dense Foods

Focus on incorporating nutrient dense foods that provide essential vitamins, minerals, and antioxidants. Here are some food groups to prioritize:

- **Proteins**: Lean meats, poultry, fish, tofu, beans, legumes, eggs, and dairy products.
- **Vegetables**: Leafy greens, cruciferous vegetables, colorful bell peppers, carrots, and sweet potatoes.
- **Fruits**: Berries, citrus fruits, apples, bananas, and melons.
- **Whole Grains**: Brown rice, quinoa, oats, barley, and whole wheat products.
- **Healthy Fats:** Avocados, nuts, seeds, olive oil, and fatty fish.

Create a Weekly Meal Plan

A well-structured weekly meal plan helps streamline the prepping process and ensures variety in your diet. Here's how to create an effective meal plan:

1. Assess Your Schedule: Identify days when you have more energy to cook and days when you might need pre prepared meals.

2. Choose Recipes: Select recipes that are easy to prepare, store well, and meet your nutritional needs. Aim for a mix of cooked meals, salads, and snacks.

3. Plan for Leftovers: Incorporate leftovers into your meal plan to minimize food waste and reduce cooking time.

4. Include Snacks: Plan for healthy snacks like yogurt, fruit, nuts, and smoothies to keep your energy levels stable throughout the day.

Make a Detailed Grocery List

Once you have your meal plan, create a detailed grocery list to ensure you have all the necessary ingredients. Group items by category (produce, dairy, grains, etc.) to make shopping more efficient. Buying in bulk can also be cost effective and reduce the frequency of shopping trips.

- Prep in Batches

Batch cooking is an excellent way to prepare multiple meals in one go. Set aside a few hours each week to cook large quantities of food that can be divided into individual portions and stored in the refrigerator or freezer. Here are some batch cooking ideas:

Soups and Stews: These are easy to make in large quantities and freeze well. Consider making vegetable soup, chicken stew, or lentil soup.

Casseroles: Dishes like lasagna, shepherd's pie, and vegetable casseroles can be made ahead of time and portioned out.

Grains and Beans: Cook a big batch of brown rice, quinoa, or beans and use them as bases for various meals throughout the week.

Proteins: Grill or bake a large quantity of chicken breasts, tofu, or fish that can be added to salads, sandwiches, or eaten as main dishes.

- Invest in Quality Storage Containers

Proper storage is crucial for maintaining the freshness and quality of your prepped meals. Invest in a set of high quality, BPA free containers in various sizes. Glass containers are an excellent option as they are durable and can be used for both storage and reheating. Label each container with the contents and date to keep track of your meals and avoid spoilage.

- Utilize Freezer Space

Freezing prepped meals is a great way to extend their shelf life and ensure you always have healthy options on hand. Here are some tips for effective freezing:

Portion Control: Divide meals into individual servings before freezing. This makes it easy to thaw only what you need.

Avoid Freezer Burn: Use airtight containers or heavy duty freezer bags to prevent freezer burn. Squeeze out as much air as possible before sealing.

Flat Freezing: For soups and stews, freeze portions in freezer bags laid flat. This saves space and speeds up the thawing process.

Labeling: Clearly label each bag or container with the contents and date to keep track of what you have in your freezer.

- Incorporate Fresh Ingredients

While meal prepping, it's essential to incorporate fresh ingredients to maintain a balanced diet. Here are some tips for adding fresh components to your prepped meals:

Salads: Prewash and chop salad ingredients but keep them separate until you're ready to eat. Store greens, toppings, and dressings in separate containers.

Fresh Fruits: Slice fruits like apples, melons, and berries ahead of time and store them in airtight containers for quick snacks or meal additions.

Herbs and Spices: Fresh herbs and spices can elevate the flavor of your meals. Add them just before serving for maximum freshness.

- Make Use of Slow Cookers and Instant Pots

Slow cookers and Instant Pots are invaluable tools for meal prepping. They allow you to cook large quantities of food with minimal effort and can keep your meals warm until you're ready to eat. Here are some meal ideas:

Slow Cooker Chili: Combine beans, ground turkey, tomatoes, and spices in the slow cooker for a hearty chili that can be portioned out for the week.

Instant Pot Rice and Beans: Cook a batch of rice and beans in the Instant Pot for a versatile base that can be used in bowls, wraps, or side dishes.

Slow Cooker Chicken: Season and cook chicken breasts in the slow cooker, then shred and use them in salads, tacos, or sandwiches.

- Healthy Snack Preparation

In addition to main meals, having healthy snacks on hand is essential for maintaining energy levels and supporting your immune system. Here are some snack prep ideas:

Energy Balls: Make a batch of energy balls with oats, nut butter, honey, and dried fruit. Store them in the refrigerator for a quick and nutritious snack.

Vegetable Sticks and Hummus: Precut vegetables like carrots, celery, and bell peppers. Pair them with individual portions of hummus.

Yogurt Parfaits: Layer Greek yogurt with fresh berries and granola in small jars for a grab and go snack.

Trail Mix: Combine nuts, seeds, and dried fruit in portioned bags for a convenient and nutrient dense snack.

Adjusting for Treatment Side Effects

Cancer treatment can cause various side effects that impact your appetite and ability to eat. Tailor your meal prep to accommodate these challenges:

- **Nausea:** Prepare bland, easy to digest foods like rice, bananas, and plain toast. Ginger tea and peppermint can also help soothe nausea.

- **Mouth Sores**: Focus on soft, nonacidic foods like mashed potatoes, oatmeal, and smoothies. Avoid spicy and crunchy foods that can irritate sores.

- **Taste Changes**: Experiment with different flavors and textures to find what is most palatable. Marinate proteins, use fresh herbs, and try citrus based dressings to enhance flavor.

Hydration

Staying hydrated is crucial, especially during cancer treatment. Incorporate hydrating foods and beverages into your meal prep:

- Infused Water: Prepare pitchers of water infused with fruits like lemon, cucumber, and berries to encourage hydration.
- Broth Based Soups: Make broths and soups that not only provide hydration but also essential nutrients.
- Smoothies: Blend fruits and vegetables with water or coconut water for a hydrating and nutritious drink.

Flexibility and Adaptation

Be flexible with your meal plans and be ready to adapt based on your energy levels, appetite, and taste preferences. It's okay to adjust recipes and meal components to better suit how you're feeling on any given day.

Seek Support

Meal prepping can be a collaborative effort. Enlist the help of family members or friends, or consider hiring a meal prep service if it's within your budget. This can alleviate some of the burdens and ensure you have a steady supply of nutritious meals.

Continual Learning and Adjustment

Meal prepping is a skill that improves with practice. Continue to learn and adjust your methods to better suit your needs. Attend workshops, read books, and seek advice from nutrition experts to enhance your meal prepping techniques.

Chapter 8: Building a Sustainable Lifestyle

Maintaining Healthy Eating Habits beyond Treatment

Cancer is difficult. There's no two ways about it. Diagnosis and treatment may be terrifying and tiring, and once you've overcome those obstacles, you'll need to adjust to life after cancer.

You may have experienced appetite loss, alterations in your perceptions of taste and smell, and episodes of nausea while undergoing cancer treatment. Eating consistently during treatment may have seemed like a chore. However, as a cancer survivor, you are likely to restore your appetite.

As you return to a more regular regimen, it's critical to keep track of what and how much you're consuming. Some survivors wish to recover weight after losing too much, whilst others may prefer to maintain or even drop a few pounds following treatment. Using the conclusion of cancer treatment as a fresh start, now is an excellent time to focus on developing healthy eating habits.

1. Eat smaller and more frequent meals

If you need to gain weight, you may not be hungry for a big meal or breakfast. Instead, fulfill your calorie needs by nibbling on nutritious meals throughout the day. Breakfast may be a hardboiled egg, followed by a banana in the middle of the morning, then a scoop of tuna salad for lunch, and so on. This method can also help you avoid overeating when attempting to lose weight.

2. Experiment with different protein sources

Proteins are the building blocks of life and an essential component of any healthy dietary plan. Proteins contribute to muscle mass gain, as well as cell repair and regeneration. Because proteins take longer to digest, eating them will keep you fuller for longer and reduce your desire for unhealthy snacks. number is the spice of life, and luckily, you can get your protein from a number of sources, including red meat, fish, eggs, tofu, almonds, beans, and cheese.

3. Avoid empty calories

You may need to eat more calories to gain weight, but not all calories are the same. Sugars and saturated fats are plentiful in calories, yet they can have harmful health consequences, as studies have repeatedly demonstrated.

Avoid consuming too much processed meals, carbs, sweets, and drinks.

4. Do not forget about fiber

Most individuals understand that dietary fiber can help prevent and relieve constipation. It also reduces cholesterol and regulates blood sugar levels. Because high fiber foods are lower in energy density than other foods, they contain less calories than low fiber ones. They are also more filling than low fiber meals, so you will feel fuller for longer after eating them. Fruits like apples and oranges, vegetables like cauliflower and green beans, whole grains like oats and wheat bran, and legumes are all good sources of fiber.

5. Use seasonings

If you still have long term therapy side effects that make eating unpleasant (such as nausea or taste alterations), season your meal to make it more appetizing. Lemon juice, cinnamon, garlic, dill, and rosemary are just a few healthful spices that may improve the flavor of dull foods. While salt is a spice, it is critical to limit the quantity of salt you consume each day to protect your heart health.

6. Try Various Food Preparations

Vegetables are vital for a well-balanced diet. If you're used to eating them one way and don't particularly enjoy them, try various methods to cook them. Veggies can be eaten crisp and raw with a nutritious dip, such seasoned Greek yogurt, steamed and topped with cheese, or chopped and mixed into soups, meatloaf, omelets, and so on. Additionally, steaming, baking, and broiling meats or fish is far healthier than frying or sautéing them.

7. Eat the rainbow

The hues of fruits and vegetables indicate the many nutrients that our bodies require. Choose fresh food in a variety of hues, such as dark leafy greens, deep yellow squash, oranges, and red peppers.

8. Shop the perimeter

Fresh foods provide the most nutritional value. When you go grocery shopping, the majority of your purchases should come from the store's perimeter. This often includes the vegetable area, meat and seafood counters, and dairy aisle. Avoid processed foods that are often packaged in cans, bags, and cartons.

Cooking Tips and Simple Recipes for Everyday Meals

When you are too tired or ill to buy food or prepare, or if you are missing meals while undergoing treatment, the following fast meal and snack suggestions may be useful. Some may not appear to be healthy options, but if you have a weak appetite, it is critical to focus on high protein, high kilojoule foods and drinks to ensure your body receives all of the necessary energy. When your hunger returns, you can resume following the healthy eating rules. Avoid meals that may exacerbate any treatment related negative effects. If you have another health problem, such as diabetes, some of the ideas may not be appropriate.

Everybody has distinct taste buds. As a caretaker, always ask your cancer patient, "What do you like to eat?" Everyone has their favorite meals and preferences. Some people are more willing to try new cuisines, while others have particular dishes they are used to. Food will go to waste if you make something that the cancer patient is unwilling to try.

Avoid your favorite meals two days before and three days after treatment. If you becomes ill while receiving chemotherapy, you may acquire food aversions to foods to which you are exposed.

Taste buds might change throughout cancer therapy. This occurs often throughout treatment. For example, dishes with very little salt may appear highly salty to someone. As a caretaker, Ask for comments, and don't take it personally if the cancer patient doesn't like what you created. This isn't about you. This is about preparing something that cancer patients can eat.

Keep the portions manageable. Cancer therapy can reduce a cancer patient's appetite. So, they are typically encouraged to consume small meals throughout the day. Looking into the refrigerator at a large batch of chicken noodle soup might be intimidating and unappealing. Use tiny containers or freezer bags to store food in reasonable snack/meal portion sizes. Label the contents and date when the dish was made. Freeze these separate pieces so that the cancer patient may take one at a time, according to their desires and hunger.

Use mineral rich broth as the soup's foundation. One of the first things to do is create a huge pot of Magic Mineral Broth or Bone Broth. This serves as the soup basis for any soups for cancer patients.

I keep quart size containers of these broths in my freezer so I can bring them out anytime I'm preparing soup.

Enrich meals naturally. Many cancer patients lose weight during treatment, therefore learnt to add calories to diets using natural substances. For example, you could add coconut oil and/or nut butters to smoothies, or use an additional tablespoon or two of extra virgin olive oil or ghee when sautéing veggies for a soup you're creating. If dairy can be allowed by the cancer patient, heavy cream can be added to pureed soups. Alternatively, coconut milk, high fat nut milk, or cream (such as Macadamia Nut Milk or Cashew Cream) can be utilized.

Eating with mouth sores and difficulties swallowing. Cancer therapy can lead to oral sores and, in some situations, trouble eating and swallowing. In these situations, having the proper consistency in meals might assist. Smoothies, pureed soups, and pureed meals are typically simpler for you to digest. The consistency should not be too thin (to prevent choking) or too thick (too difficult to swallow). If you develops mouth sores, try to avoid hot and acidic foods (for example, ginger and tomatoes). Furthermore, cold or room temperature foods are typically simpler to consume.

Eating despite sickness. Nausea is one of the most common reasons you avoid eating. Although anti-nausea medicine can assist, some people have extreme nausea and are unable to eat for an extended length of time. Drinking nourishing broth throughout the day might help. A cancer patient requested this Lemongrass Ginger Chicken Broth with fine egg noodles on a weekly basis since she was having difficulties swallowing food. Each cancer patient is unique, so it may take some experimentation to determine what is most easily tolerated.

- Light Meal and Drink Ideas

Light Meals

- Baked beans on toast with grated cheese Toasted crumpets or muffins with cheese and fruit
- Scrambled or poached eggs on toast with a glass of orange juice.
- Tuna or sardines on buttered bread with fresh tomato
- Breakfast options include an omelet with cheese or mushrooms and buttered bread, or toast with cheese, avocado, or peanut butter, topped with sliced banana and yogurt.
- Cereal or toasted muesli served with full cream milk and yogurt.

- Porridge or rice pudding with milk and cream.
- Congee Pancakes or French toast with fruit and maple syrup.

Nourishing beverages

- Enriched milk combined with AktaVite, milo, or Horlicks
- Banana smoothie
- Mango lassi
- Hot chocolate
- Flavored milk
- Apricot lemon crush

Main meal ideas

- Fresh or frozen fish with chips and salad Grilled lamb cutlets, mashed potato with margarine or butter, and peas and carrots
- Pasta with readymade sauce, such as pesto or bolognaise, and cheese.
- Cheesy Vegetable Bake
- Options for meals include lentil dhal with chapatis or rice, green or red chicken or veggie curry with basmati rice, and salmon, tuna, or egg with store bought mayonnaise, salad, and buttered bread roll.

- Fresh or frozen lasagna or moussaka.

- Options include frittata or quiche, as well as salmon or tofu with soba noodles.

- Microwave potatoes with baked beans and cheese.

- Egg, tempeh, and sautéed veggies with gado gado (peanut) dressing.

- Wrap in falafel, hummus, and salad.

- Occasional takeout such as noodles, stir fry, curry and rice, hamburgers, or pizza (provided the meal is freshly cooked).

- Refrigerated leftover meals from the previous day; reheat till steaming.

Snack Ideas

Optional snacks include cheese crackers, pita bread with hummus, buttered pikelets, scones, muffins, fruit buns, crumpets, finger buns, and raisin toast.

- Celery with cream cheese or peanut butter.

- Hard cooked eggs.

- Dried fruits and nuts.

- Jaffles, sandwiches, and toast; try egg and store bought mayonnaise, cheese, peanut butter, avocado, canned salmon or tuna.

- Milk puddings, such as creamed rice, rice pudding, custard, mousse and quick puddings

- Fruit (fresh, frozen, stewed, or canned) with custard, yogurt, jelly, ice cream, cream, or condensed milk.

- Creamy soup with extra cream and buttered bread

- Hot fries, fish fingers, or chicken nuggets

- Instant noodles with frozen veggies

- Potato crisps, pretzels, or corn chips with dips like salsa or guacamole

- Yogurt or ice cream frozen sausage rolls, meat pies, samosas, or spring rolls.

Implementing these meal and snack options into your daily routine, you can ensure that you are obtaining enough nutrients to support your body during treatment, even on days when you don't feel well. Adjust these ideas to suit your unique tastes and tolerance levels, and always seek individualized guidance from your healthcare specialist.

Maintaining a Positive Mindset and Celebrating Achievements

Maintaining a positive mindset during cancer treatment is essential for your emotional and physical wellbeing. It's easy to feel overwhelmed by the challenges, but finding ways to stay positive and celebrating small achievements can significantly impact your journey.

In 2022, Dave celebrated what he calls his fourth birthday—four years since his transplant and being cancer-free. It's been four years since he got his life back. However, there were times when it was difficult for Dave to picture being here, happy and healthy, and enjoying life again.

When Dave was originally diagnosed with Acute Myeloid Leukemia (AML), he wanted to know everything: what the blood counts meant, what the medications were called, why he was taking them, and how the treatment was impacting his blood counts. He was really analytical, and he grew captivated by his body and the science and biology behind it all.

Dave believes people want to know all the specifics because understanding the blood levels and what is going on helps them feel a little more in control.

"When you get AML, one of your first thoughts is, 'What do I need to do to beat this?' What can be done, and how can I support it?"

This is where the majority of Dave's ambitions originated. Doctors informed him that even the tiniest workouts in his hospital room would assist, so he set a target of 30 sit-to-stands every day, which he gradually increased over time.

Dave had a really painful mouth after the treatment, so when he was given a mouthwash that could be used up to 20 times per day, he made sure to take all 20 doses! Even with the moisturizer they prescribed to care for his skin, he set a goal to apply it a particular number of times each day.

If there was ever anything said that could assist him, he would take it. Maybe it was his competitive nature or his desire to be in control, but it got him through.

Dave's family also helped him find his mission. His family had lost several folks to cancer. Dave lost his uncle Andy to cancer not long before he was diagnosed, and he was quite close to Andy's sons.

So it was motivating for him to deviate from the norm for them—to be a beacon of something unique. That was his main focus during treatment.

"But how can you be positive when you're going through this arduous therapy and wherever you look, there's a new side effect or a new piece of information from the physicians that raises concerns?"

Dave and his wife were both obsessed with viewing encouraging films and hearing success stories from other people with AML. They wanted to see genuine people at the other end of the road, living proof that it was possible. This absolutely motivated Dave; he was eager for it and actively sought it out.

AML success rate data? Dave was uninterested in them since they did not benefit him. He was going to get through this in his own manner. Other people's success stories inspired him to believe he could achieve it.

The second major thing Dave did to shift his viewpoint was to actively combat the idea in his brain that chemo was a poison and that the therapy was the enemy. Cancer is the adversary. Chemotherapy is your medication.

It's recognized for being a combination of extremely powerful medications, poisonous, and harmful to the body—but it may be beneficial if it works! Chemotherapy is a frightening term, yet it is truly excellent, even lifesaving.

"When I was having extremely acute rigidity and my legs were trembling so much, my doctor stated, 'Just consider what it's doing to leukemia—your likelihood of relapse is now reduced because of this treatment.'"

Of course, no one has perfect control over the result of their therapy, but we can influence how we see things.

"For example, can you be proud of yourself? When you have AML, you may find yourself completing a variety of medical tasks that you were previously unaware of, like caring for your PICC line or dealing with side effects. It's difficult to deal with all of this without medical training, therefore you should acknowledge your own strengths."

Dave feels proud right now. He is proud to be on the other side, to be a champion for the NHS, and to share his experience to aid others. Knowing he has this strength within him, he believes it will stay with him forever and guide him through life. All he wants now is to live a happy life with his family.

Also, from Dave's story, you can draw inspiration and strength regardless of the type of cancer you are battling.

Every cancer journey is unique, but maintaining a positive mindset and celebrating achievements are universally powerful strategies. Whether you are dealing with AML, breast cancer, lung cancer, or any other type, the principles remain the same. Focus on what you can control, set small, achievable goals, and find joy in the little victories. Lean on your support system, whether it's family, friends, or healthcare providers, and seek out stories of hope and success. These narratives can inspire and remind you that you are not alone in this fight.

Remember, your mindset can significantly influence your journey. Viewing treatment as a tool for healing rather than an adversary can make a substantial difference in your outlook and overall wellbeing. Celebrate every milestone, no matter how small, and acknowledge your strength and resilience. This positive approach will not only enhance your quality of life but also provide the motivation needed to face each day with courage and determination. Your journey is one of strength, hope, and continuous progress.

As you near the end of your trip through **Optimal Nutrition for Cancer Patients**, it becomes obvious that the power of food extends beyond just sustaining your bodies. It's about empowerment, healing, and celebrating tiny triumphs along the path. The appropriate nutrition may be a powerful friend in your battle against cancer, boosting your immune system, managing side effects, and improving your overall quality of life.

Remember that this book is only a guide, a starting point. Your journey is unique, so listen to your body, seek assistance from your healthcare team, and be adaptable in your approach. Celebrate your accomplishments, no matter how minor, and be optimistic as you move forward.

Stay informed, motivated, and most importantly, optimistic. Together, we can pave the way to greater health, one nutritious meal at a time. Here to your fortitude, resilience, and quest to health.

Thank You!

Dear Reader,

Thank you for joining me on this journey through **Optimal Nutrition for Cancer Patients**. Your time, attention, and dedication to learning about the powerful role of nutrition in cancer care mean the world to me. I hope this book has provided you with valuable insights, practical advice, and a sense of empowerment as you navigate your health journey.

As a token of my appreciation, I'm offering you a special gift: a downloadable meal planning guide and groceries shopping list filled with additional recipes, tips, and resources to support you in maintaining a nutritious and balanced diet. I hope this gift continues to aid you in your journey towards better health and well-being.

If you found this book helpful, I kindly ask you to leave a review on Amazon and rate my book. Your feedback is incredibly valuable and helps others discover the benefits of nutritional guidance in cancer care. Sharing your thoughts and experiences can make a significant difference in the lives of others facing similar challenges.

Once again, thank you for allowing me to be a part of your journey. Wishing you strength, health, and happiness.

Warm regards,

Johanne M. Martinez